Praise for Michael Harding

'Harding is a self-deprecating and winsome writer
whose bittersweet musings on middle-age, loneliness
and the search for spiritual enlightenment . . . are
leavened by an incredibly dry and unforced wit'
Metro Herald

'Often funny, occasionally disturbing and
not without its moments of deep sadness,
Harding has peeled back his soul and held it
out on the palm of his hand for all to see'
Christine Dwyer-Hickey

'A repository of modern man's deepest fears,
Harding emerges as something of an embattled
hero for our times . . . It's rare for a memoir to
demand such intense emotional involvement,
and rarer still for it to be so fully rewarded'
Sunday Times

'Hilarious, and tender, and mad, and harrowing, and wistful, and always beautifully written. A wonderful book'
Kevin Barry

'Beautifully written . . . gives us permission to be lost, sick, sad, creative, happy and compassionate – in short, to be human'
Mary McEvoy, *Irish Independent*

'This memoir grabs you from the outset and holds you right to the end. His language sings'
Deirdre Purcell

'Written in lyrical prose, it provides a compelling insight into the turbulent emotions that rage behind so many of the bland faces we meet in everyday life'
Sunday Business Post

'This frank and unflinching memoir offers a fascinating insight into the mind of the author of two of the finest Irish novels of the eighties'
Pat McCabe

'Difficult to put down'
The Irish Times

Michael Harding is an author and playwright. A recipient of the Stewart Parker Award for theatre, a Hennessy Award for Short Stories and a Bank of Ireland/RTÉ award for Excellence in the Arts in 1990, he has written numerous plays for the Abbey Theatre and was writer in association with the National Theatre in 1993.

He is a member of Aosdána, a columnist for over fifteen years with *The Irish Times* and his podcasts are available on the Patreon platform.

Also by Michael Harding

Non-fiction

All the Things Left Unsaid
A Cloud Where the Birds Rise
(with Jacob Stack)
What Is Beautiful in the Sky
Chest Pain
On Tuesdays I'm a Buddhist
Talking to Strangers
Hanging with the Elephant
Staring at Lakes

Fiction

Bird in the Snow
The Trouble with Sarah Gullion
Priest

MICHAEL HARDING

I Loved Him From The Day He Died

HACHETTE
BOOKS
IRELAND

First published in Ireland in 2024 by
HACHETTE BOOKS IRELAND

1

The title of this book has been adapted from a line in 'Death of an
Irishwoman' by Michael Hartnett from *Collected Poems* (2001) and is used
with the kind permission of the Author's Estate and The Gallery Press.

This book includes an adapted piece on David Marcus, which was first
published in *David Marcus: Editing Ireland* (2024), edited by Paul Delaney
and Deirdre Madden and published by The Stinging Fly Press.

Illustrations: Nick Ellwood.

Cataloguing in Publication Data is available from the British Library

ISBN: 9781529379228

Typeset in Minion Pro by Palimpsest Book Production Ltd, Falkirk, Stirlingshire

Printed and bound in Great Britain by Clays Ltd, Elcograf, S.p.A.

Hachette Books Ireland policy is to use papers that are natural, renewable
and recyclable products and made from wood grown in sustainable
forests. The logging and manufacturing processes are expected to
conform to the environmental regulations of the country of origin.

Hachette Books Ireland
8 Castlecourt Centre
Castleknock
Dublin 15, Ireland

A division of Hachette UK Ltd
Carmelite House, 50 Victoria Embankment, EC4Y 0DZ

www.hachettebooksireland.ie

For Joe and Annie

Contents

PART TWO

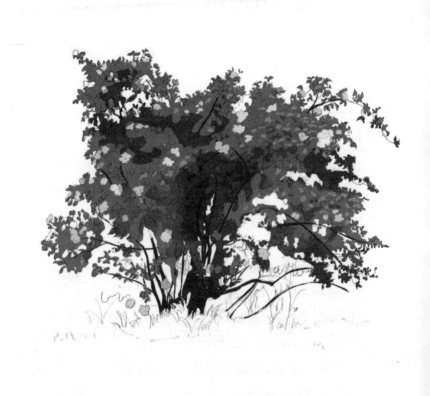

A Pilgrimage Is Like Life; it Is About Letting Go

On the sixth of August in 2023 I was seventy years old. And I asked myself how I ended up at the back of the house in a shed overlooking the lake. In fact, it's a very large garden room behind the house, cluttered with religious paraphernalia.

Outside this room time moves slowly. My beloved comes and goes on the pathway through the garden to her studio where another universe spins in its own cosmic mysteries. And occasionally my daughter arrives, in a jeep, all smiles and full of stories about horses.

The cats pace across the backyard looking for dinner. One of them is blind, one of them has a broken back, and the king tom is black and moves like a lion. We call him Charlie. He is our favourite. He almost died ten years ago by swallowing the bone of a chicken leg. I saw it going into his mouth. I was watching from the window. But it was too late to stop him. It was going in and down his gullet like he loved it. The vet gave him tablets that softened the bone inside and it turned to a kind of cement in his stomach and ever since he has suffered occasionally from a light bleed. But I suppose compared to my own gut, which hasn't functioned smoothly in a decade, he got off lightly. So, life goes on in the yard outside and everything out there is dramatic, and everything in here is quiet.

Like a womb, with a warm stove in winter, and background music from a sound bar, and I sit dozing by the fire all day. But now I realise my entire life has slipped away in this refuge and that worries me.

And if not in this room, then in other rooms like it. One studio after another. All because I am a writer. In the studio there is no time. It's a continuous moment into which I step again and again on each new day. A place where the stove is always lit, the little flames flicker in the grate and the cast-iron box throws out a fiercely comforting heat. I sit on a soft armchair listening to Brahms or Beethoven, or some *sean-nós* singer, or the All-Night Vespers of Rachmaninoff.

And although I've written about my mother, and my childhood, and my beloved, and the cats and the trees and wild horses, I have never written about my father.

So, on my seventieth birthday I resolved to walk a short Camino in Spain sometime during the following twelve months: from Sarria to Santiago, echoing the pilgrims of history that made the journey to hear the great bell and see the magnificent thurible swing across the sanctuary in the cathedral dedicated to the apostle James.

I told nobody what my intention was. I was worried that people might think it was a silly idea. Sentimental and indulgent. To walk with my father on the Camino. I just said I'd like to stretch my legs a little.

My father was forty-seven years dead in 2023. Almost half a century. So that may have been a trigger. And I hoped some part of him would be with me. I could ponder his story, reflect on his life, think about his character. I could resolve the mystery of how I relate to him, and he to me, and what it means to have a father.

Maybe it was also because I was seventy and had been through a few minor illnesses and this was an end-of-life yearning in me. An awakening appropriate for someone touching old age. A bucket-list priority: to make a pilgrimage, and to know my father.

Although, to be honest, it worried me that I might not be physically fit for the full walk so I chose to book a trip that would allow me six days to complete 126 kilometres. They told me that was the easy Camino.

Demons whispered in my ear that it was a waste of time and that if I had not resolved my relationship with my father by now, it wasn't likely that walking the laneways of Spain was going to change anything. But nonetheless I began to embrace the idea that I would walk the holy pathway, and in the end, I would be a different person by the time I got to the cathedral in the city of Santiago. Even if I did not come to know my father better, at least the pilgrimage might make me a better person. Although any therapist might have told me this was magical thinking and far too much to expect.

I have worked with a therapist on several occasions through the years. Because in the past I have suffered from anxiety and have lived like a prisoner in my studio.

The road to Santiago is wonderful because it is not just a geographical fact. The pathway floats in the imaginal realm. The road to Santiago is a road to everywhere. You walk through the decades of your life, you meet the people you loved both living and dead, and in the end, you find that just physically walking has brought your mind into the heart, and your heart has once again become the compass of life.

At a surface level it is a pathway to a city in the province of Galicia in northern Spain. But in the imaginal realm it is also a journey towards the Buddha, and it is the meandering medieval track of many a bewildered saint. In short, like any pilgrim way, it is a journey at the physical level and a journey into the interior of the mind. I might be a poet in search of the moon, or a child going home to Mother. These are possibilities open to anyone. Because the Camino is for everyone.

Although never once did I think of it as a child going home to Daddy. That was a frame of intimacy that never quite existed in my childhood so how could it surface in the narrative of old age? A recollection of walking or running towards Daddy long ago doesn't exist and I don't remember any such spontaneous moment in childhood. It is like I never knew him. And yet that was the purpose of the pilgrimage. To discover him where he might still reside inside me.

But as I sat in my studio, comforted by Christian icons, the Mother of God, Christ of Sinai, three wise men, Jacob, Nicodemus and Irenaeus whom I found in a car boot sale in Carrick-on-Shannon, and a view of the lake, flicking through brochures from U Walk, a travel company in Navan, I never imagined my father would come so close to me as he did on the road to Santiago.

I dreamed of a perfect pilgrimage. I dreamed I was sitting at a window on a hot night in Spain, where the cicadas sing and the wine bottle on the table is empty and the smell of fresh bread fills the room and a girl with brown hair and berry-brown skin is eating olives and her rucksack lies in the corner, the shell of Compostela hanging from the straps, and us talking maybe about her father or my father or the one Father in all of us.

'Just imagine if my father was your father,' I say to her, and then I wake with a shock.

'What's wrong with you?' the beloved asks. 'Can you not sleep?'

'I keep thinking of the Camino,' I say, hiding almost everything.

On the train to Dublin one day I met an old monk. He boarded the train in Mullingar, an elderly man in a brown Franciscan habit and brown sandals. He sat opposite me and stared so long into my face that he frightened the wits out of me. A no-nonsense kind of monk. Perhaps he's just an old man with a short fuse, I thought. Not grumpy but volatile.

I told him how I was going to do the Camino in Spain during the spring or summer. I thought that might impress him. It didn't.

He just sneered and stared and so I avoided him for the rest of the journey by looking at my phone and staring out the window. To my relief he rose to leave as the train pulled into Maynooth station. I watched the high walls of the seminary that skirted the train tracks. I could see the spire and the rooftops of the dormitories within. Rooms I had spent years in while studying for the priesthood in my twenties. The spire of the great chapel where I had prostrated before the altar to be ordained. Avenues on the far side of the wall where I had walked year in and year out in the hope of finding some kind of fatherly God.

That was my seminary life, which my father in Cavan funded though he disapproved of it. On my first year he tried to persuade me to do something else. So much so that after a year I left the seminary, continued as a lay student until I had completed my Bachelor of Arts degree and then went in search of an alternative career as a teacher in Glangevlin. Only after he died in July of 1976 did I write to the authorities in Maynooth asking them if they would allow me to resume my studies in the seminary.

The old monk grabbed a briefcase from the rack overhead and leaned down to say something to me.

'Don't forget that a pilgrimage is like life; it is all about letting go.'

And suddenly I woke and realised he was only a creature in my dreaming. I was dozing on the train. But we were indeed slowing down, approaching the station in Maynooth. And sure enough there was a quiet little man in brown robes opposite me who I thought gave me a strange look before he disembarked.

PART ONE

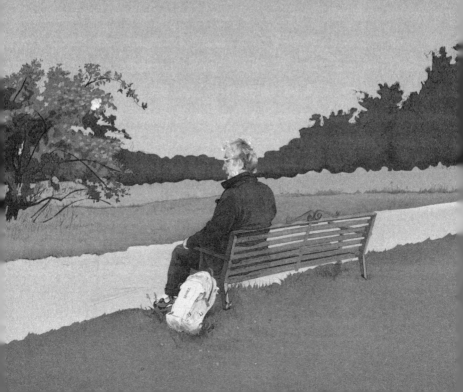

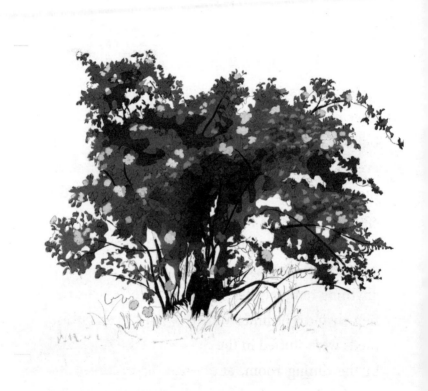

A Stranger in the Fog

I spent years in public houses, both before and after my father died, not for the sake of libation but because I was at some level searching for him everywhere – from public houses to quiet sanctuaries, and in books I wrote and beneath the spotlight in every public hall and theatre.

Not that he was in any way an heroic figure; even before his death he had drifted far away from anything remotely like 'my daddy'. Because he was fiercely old. His limbs were ivory, his constipation meds were stuffed in the drawers of the sideboard in the dining room, and whatever occupied his mind as he stretched on his bed listening to BBC Radio 3 was not anything I might understand.

Every time I saw him in those feeble moments, reclining on beds or asleep on a deckchair, I despised him a little. What kind of father would just lie there doing nothing? What daddy could dare to be so old?

Going to the pub was an alternative reality. Meeting men was a metaphor. Every old man was, as the poem says, my father. And I embodied the metaphor as I stood at the counter of each new bar.

It began the moment I stepped into a pub on Main Street in Cavan. I was sixteen. I brushed up against older men for the first time with a new intimacy. I smoked Major cigarettes. I ordered pints and held a half-crown out in my sweaty boyish palm. I was sure that I had become a man on that occasion.

There was hardly enough space for a single row of drinkers at the bar. People sat on high stools, shoulder to shoulder, and along the wall behind them there was a ledge where another row of customers stood. The space was more like a corridor to nowhere.

Sometimes poets in their twenties would arrive, bearded men with loose tobacco and hip flasks of whiskey, and girls in dungarees following beside them, all aglow with their boyfriends' boldness.

Civil servants got plastered on high stools. Teachers in the secondary schools were addressed with first-name intimacy by young fellows they had once chastised in class. Everyone was squashed together, and mostly male. And as clear as the billowing smoke of our cigarettes, a blue fog of loneliness enveloped us in a patriarchal barracks.

But it had what every Irish pub can promise above all else – a sense of belonging and intimacy; and those were the things I never had with my father.

Somewhere in that world of broken masculinity I could smell my father. As if he was there and not in the dining room at home where he sat with his shirt sleeves rolled up and his braces holding up the trousers of his blue suit as he tackled an evening salad of lettuce, ham, boiled egg and a few slices of a tomato as hard as a turnip. He was not at home any longer. He was there among the bleary-eyed ones, the old men drenched in remorse and the working-class boys with supple bodies from physical labour. Because of his age and remoteness, his gentility and discretion became a shadow on the floor. A trace of smoke in the air. A shaft of sunlight slicing through blue plumes of smoke above our heads. It all blended into a blur of laughter and beer stains and cigarette ash on the floor, and I could almost reach out and grasp something in the air and say, 'It's you, Daddy, isn't it?' Here, surely, in this mob, in this aching collection of sorrow, you must be here, Daddy!

Maybe he was there watching me? In the shadow of the public house? Waiting for me in the wings of the stage as I finished a performance?

There was a kind of hole at the centre of every bar, lounge or bawdy party that I stepped into, and it became so enormous that the world got swallowed by emptiness

His gift as a father was his gentle and remote wisdom. But his failure was his lack of intimacy. The burden that I carried as he grew old was the void in him. Even before his death I felt I had failed to find belonging with him, and that he belonged nowhere.

That's how tethered I remained over many years to the man in Cavan who sat under his standard lamp during my childhood. And the void he left in the heart filled up with a longing for him.

There was tenderness in him certainly when he tried to hug or kiss me goodnight, or when he tried to explain, when he was resting on the bed listening to Radio 3, that he was really thinking of heaven and how it might be just like the beauty of this life except more magnified. And there must have been much more tenderness evident long ago in all the songs he once sang, and which people remembered him singing at parties many years before I was born. But that tenderness passed me by. I didn't feel it.

He couldn't quite do the physical things that daddies do. Maybe he had no emotional intelligence at all, and so could not communicate how he felt apart from just talking his emotions down the phone. And if I ached for it as a child when he was alive, then my body surely screeched out for it as a man, when after the funeral I found that he was gone and had left this gap, this space of nothing inside me which could only be filled with a clatter of masculinity, sweat and beer, and which was promised at the door of every public house in the country.

After the funeral I found myself remembering snippets of his story as he had filtered it for me over the years of my childhood. His own father's romantic love for a girl that worked in a hat shop on Cuffe Street in Dublin, and the consequent marriage and the birth of two children in the Guinness Buildings in Dublin's Liberties, a home for destitutes. And then his mother's death when he and his sister were still infants, and their impoverished childhood in a two-room cottage on Beaver Row in Donnybrook, with his Polish grandmother, her two sons and two grandchildren. And then his sister's death.

He gave me fragmented images of an Uncle Samuel who played music on a mouth harp and did turns in music halls. But I could never tell the whole story. I could never say why his mother died so young. Why he was born in poverty. Why his father was useless. And where on the Lithuanian/Polish border his granny may have come from. Because he never offered any details.

There were terrible gaps. And then he died. And it was over.

Sometimes his story welled up inside me and became my story. His father taking him to every new play at the Abbey Theatre during the turbulent years after 1916 shimmered inside me as a memory, when I walked the same streets after watching some play of my own in that same Abbey Theatre. His Uncle Samuel dancing on the flags of the little kitchen in Donnybrook. His grandmother and her sister drinking punch at Christmas when they met to remember their long-ago lives in Poland.

Such colour and fun and theatre, and yet all I knew was an accountant who lived in the drawing room and was terrified that the tiny minds of the local middle classes would turn against him if they knew of his impoverished background.

Even the memory of him in braces and shirt, at sixty years of age, holding a spade in his soft little hands, the sun blinding him despite the shades that he clipped onto his thick lenses when he was outside, filled me with sympathy for his fragile body and his jam-jar-bottom spectacles and his white chicken limbs. It all left a kind of emptiness and longing for something stronger, more muscular and male. He filled me with this 'nothingness' when I yearned to be a man.

In my late teens and early twenties, I drank all over the country when I was loose on the roads in summertime, thinking maybe that he might be curious, or ask me where I had been the night before, or where I was going when I went away for two weeks on the trot. But rural Ireland beyond the drawing room was a jungle to him.

'I'm going to stay with a friend,' I'd say. 'He's in my class in Maynooth.' And I'd hitch lifts to Derry or Cork to visit classmates.

Yet in another way, he came with me; my father was like a ghost beside me even as I stood on ditches and waited in hope for the next car to pass. No more than a shadow beneath a signpost or a figure in a black coat at the far end of a bar. I accepted him like one accepts a river or a mountain.

The father inside me.

I would compare every car I hitched to my father's Austin A40. Was it bigger? Flashier?

Smaller? And every driver that I shared a cigarette with had arms I scrutinised, maybe bronze from working in the fields, and I'd think of my poor little daddy and his ridiculous limbs.

But now as I sit by the fire in my studio and look back on those days more than fifty years ago, I am broken-hearted and remorseful that I wasted so much time in this little room. Too many years spent alone and melancholic, wasting time by reflecting on the passing of time. Too much time being a writer, which is what he made of me.

I fumbled around for many years because I wanted him to be someone he wasn't. I wanted me to be someone I wasn't. I didn't know that his need for belonging was my need for belonging.

I spent a lifetime trying to find him but only when small illnesses prefigured the ultimate destination of my own human life was I released from the expectations I had put on him. I wanted him to be the source of my being, the foundation of my meaning, the homeland where I belonged. But he was none of those things. He was just a man.

I see all those nights from the past as they flit by in my memory. One pub after another, one bar after another. An endless longing for company and fun and craic that propelled me through the doors of so many lounges, snugs and function rooms in hundreds of hotels.

And what was I looking for?

It might have been reassurance, some endorsement of who I was as a man. An endorsement of masculinity, perhaps. Other times it may have been healing that I was looking for in the face of all the self-loathing that arises not just in childhood or adolescence but throughout life when we do wrong things to others and don't know how to fix them.

What I didn't realise was that my father was a ghost in every room. Not just the feeble old man who lived in his armchair, but ever-present; a template of fatherhood as mysterious, demanding and forgiving.

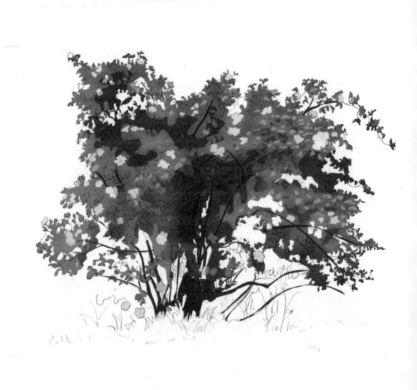

Refuge

I live near the townland of Tearmon in Leitrim, and I once created a work for Siamsa, the National Folk Theatre, called *Tearmon*, and there is hardly a county in Ireland where I have not found the word 'tearmon' or 'termon' on local signposts. The word denotes a sanctuary or boundary, marking land belonging to monks and churches wherein there was a right of sanctuary. Tearmon is a sanctuary, a place of refuge, and there are many refuges in the Irish wilderness.

But I used the word flagrantly and without discrimination. If I stepped into a cosy bar I would find the word 'refuge' surfacing in my mind. If I made a pilgrimage to some holy well in Ballyvourney or Killybegs, or to the holy wells of saints like Lazar or Ailbe on the slopes of Kilronan mountain beside me, or especially to the quiet stone structure in Ballinaglera sheltered by lovely holly and willow trees, I might say to myself that this is a moment of refuge.

A place of refuge.

Because I was always seeking that safe space in the world that is not quite of the world. The still centre of the moving circle. The sanctuary of peace in the troubled earth. That wasn't an unusual quest. It is the adventure that humans have been on ever since they became conscious: to find peace at the heart of things, to find heaven in the ordinary things.

I certainly found peace at the lip of many a holy well. But I also found it in the sleepy bars where a stove in the corner held a flame that flickered as defiantly as the sanctuary lamp in any church and where the men like old monks sighed over their pints and said nothing, discussed nothing, heard nothing and thought nothing.

That's what is both comical and wonderful about men. They can hold a space of emptiness for a long time. I can't say it any better than this: it's the hole where God used to be and perhaps where God still is.

The vacant mind. The empty streets. The silent house. That's where my father was. That's how I remember him in the drawing room, under his standard lamp, with nothing but the sound of the paper moving in his hands emanating from the room.

It was an empty space in him that attracted me. An empty space I felt in myself. The father in his solitude was the solitude in me.

My relationship with him moved through various phases over the years. I hovered at the edge of his mysterious presence when I was a child. Then as I grew, I saw his flaws and imperfections, his fragile old body; I fled to find refuge elsewhere, only to find his ghost haunting me for years. And even when I flung myself into the fun of living and drinking, showing off and performing, there was always a feeling that anything I did was not original but somehow a shadow of the template he had carried and passed on to me.

No time more clearly than when I looked in the mirror, which was nauseating. That I grew old myself was undeniable. But that I saw in each phase of my ageing the father in me emerge once again was outrageous. I could never escape him.

When I looked into the well, on the other hand, I saw nothing. That's the nature of a well. You stand at the edge so you can't see your own image. All you can see is the clear living water and the stones at the bottom. Maybe that is the tenderness of the well that draws people towards it and leads them to believe that in its water there is healing and empowerment.

It was at holy wells that I often felt most tenderly towards my father. I don't know why. The desolation of the wilder landscape can sometimes feel like love. The reeds on the shoreline sometimes sing of a homeland. In those invisible spaces, nesting near the lake shores or at some holy well, I found his presence again; and in those moments I felt his heart was like the lion, and me a lonely traveller looking for him.

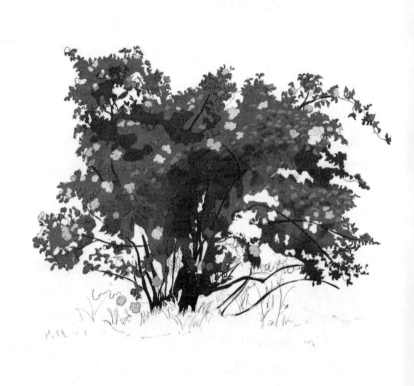

The Heart Is a Lonely Hunter

My father was sometimes aloof and distant so that I could never learn from him how to be in the world. I suspect he had many anxieties about the fragility of his body, his poor eyesight and his lack of teeth.

My father had no teeth at all. He wore enormous and crude dentures, and my mother once remarked that it was something to do with his impoverished upbringing and lack of nutrition that caused disease to set in early and so his entire set of teeth had to be removed. When I saw him in bed or in hospital, without the dentures or glasses, it was like looking at a different person. The glasses and dentures gave him a face. But without them he was deprived even of that identity, and I truly didn't know who it was lying in the bed.

He may have had other pain, not least to do with the mother he never knew, and the cut and thrust of life selling newspapers on the streets of Dublin as a child, or the life of a county accountant in Cavan trying to hide the fact that he was once a newspaper boy on the streets. Life is complicated. He died before I had time to resolve anything.

And after he died, I searched for someone I could call Daddy, in vain, poring over memories of summer holidays, Christmas dinners and family parties.

But he was always in another room, reading the paper, listening to the wireless, or sitting in the car outside some relatives' house in Dublin or Castlepollard when the rest of us were inside enjoying family fun.

What was it about his aloof presence that I could never pin down to something intimate or human? I can't say. I even tried to find him in old church records and graveyards, on ancestry.com and in book reviews he wrote for *The Irish Press*. But he remained a mystery, an enigma and an absence.

I tried to figure out where his Polish grandmother fitted in and why he retained the receipts of her burial in a Church of Ireland graveyard in Dublin, along with the Star of David, a silver pendant with the word 'Mazel' written in Hebrew at the centre, which I can only presume belonged to her. It would have been comforting if I could have found a trace of Jewish history, a drop of Jewish blood in him, obliterated perhaps because his grandmother feared shame if her ancestry was revealed. But how lonely it must have been for him, no matter who his granny was, to hold onto that pendant and the receipt of her burial location for a lifetime and remain silent on the matter.

You might say he must have been ambitious to drag himself up from squalor to become a professional in the middle classes with a house in suburbia. In fact, the only time I saw him fired by a passion for his work was when he was writing book reviews for David Marcus in *The Irish Press*. He would bend over a small table in his bedroom, on weekends or bank holidays, his jacket off and his sleeves rolled up, with the braces of his trousers strapped across his shoulders and his thick spectacles on the end of his nose as he wrote almost reverently with his fountain pen, making notes from the book he was reviewing.

'I would have loved to have been a writer,' he said sometimes, but I sensed it wasn't writing or anything else that drove him.

He didn't have ambition. And I think it was fear that nested deep inside. Fear of what he had been born into. Fear of the smells in a small house, the outdoor lavatory, the poor food, the steam from clothes steeping in an iron bathtub at the back door.

Fear of poverty made him cautious of everything and everyone. Maybe that was his real secret. That he was afraid. Although even that is still conjecture.

In every search for him, and every emotional reaching out into the dark to find him, I came up against a blank wall.

An absence.

I brooded over his poverty as a child, his determination to pull his life together, but I could never find him in the dust that was left behind. He was a ghost haunting me down the years no matter how much he led me on pathways that were echoes of his own life, as I became the clone of something I never knew.

He died in '76 but it was only when my mother died in 2012 and I was doing a final sweep of the house before selling it that I found the receipt for his grandmother's burial and the location of her grave. Attached to it was the silver pendant displaying Hebrew lettering inside a Star of David.

On the one hand, he hid himself not just from me but from the world I grew up in. And on the other hand, he left clues on a shelf for someone to find after he was gone. I will always wonder if the silver pendant was discarded by him and then forgotten, and if my discovery of it was a quirky accident of history. Did he remember that pendant in his final hours as he thought of his will and his house insurance and his bank accounts, wanting everything resolved; did he reach out for his grandmother, who in effect mothered him, just like everyone calls to their mother as they pass away?

I can never know the answers. In life he was mysterious and elusive, cold yet sensitive. Sometimes he was even tyrannical in a gentle way when it came to who boiled his eggs or how strong he liked his tea brewed. Yet they said he was a charmer in his younger days, a man who sang satirical songs ridiculing Hitler and told jokes at parties in the town before I was born.

I could never piece it all together. And on his bookshelf, I found Teilhard de Chardin, Thomas Merton, Ethel Mannin, Hilaire Belloc, G.K. Chesterton and Cardinal Newman; people who had clung to Catholic faith though they had come from elsewhere; strangers in their new-found religion. Exiles seeking refuge in a new faith or figures from the church who had been exiled. He had been very curious about outsiders.

When I went to the seminary for the first time, he sent me cut-outs from newspapers advertising jobs in the civil service.

'You might be better to try this for a while before you consider a life in the clergy,' he wrote.

A remote figure, a reclusive patriarch living alone in a drawing room with his radio and newspapers, while my brother and I endured adolescence without maps or safe places to hide, and his wife endured a kind of constrained decorum in the kitchen and liberated herself eventually by learning to drive a car as he drifted into ill health.

His aloof presence was never more obvious than when we went to visit my mother's relatives, most usually her sister, who had a public house in Castlepollard. This ancient premises was where my grandmother had come from and where my mother and her sisters had often spent their summer holidays. They'd lived in heaven during the long warm evenings, hanging around the town square and talking to boys.

When I was growing up that public house was a place of joy and wonder. An old lady we called Auntie Nellie sat in the corner of the kitchen beside the range burning with turf from the bog that my mother and her sisters had often worked on when they were teenagers. My mother and her sisters would sit for hours at the kitchen table, drinking tea from china cups neatly arranged on their dainty saucers, devouring chocolate eclairs and poring over memories of their times on the train from Cavan, and the pony and trap adventures to Sunday mass, and the days they helped the beautiful boys drive cattle through the town square to their milking parlours long, long ago. There was Nancy, a tiny bird-like woman who lived in Dublin, and Bernadette, a worrier who owned the pub, and sometimes Molly from Cavan who would look wistfully at the piano that she had played long ago at parties on wintry nights of snow during the Christmas holidays when they were all children.

It was a perfect heaven to remember and I loved the way they could fall into their old accents and girly talk, and I could sit listening to them in that kitchen for hours.

But where was my father at those moments, those tiny gatherings of casual joy that might have renewed him if he had cared to share?

The truth is that he remained outside. Auntie Bernie, as we called her, would greet her sisters and their husbands, her nieces and nephews, with cheeky kisses as we all arrived in different cars from Cavan, Dublin or Drumavaddy and then we all went inside, through the bar and down a long corridor to the kitchen at the back of the premises. But he remained outside.

Uncle Bill, Nancy's husband, a Dubliner who chain-smoked and drank whiskey in the bar and who had lungs that were forever on the verge of exhaustion, would call my father Mick.

'Are you not having a drink, Mick?' he'd say in a strong accent, and my father would shudder and say he had just come in to use the bathroom. He was the only person I knew who called my father Mick and I wondered if that might have been the reason for my father refusing to remain at the bar. But one thing is certain: for whatever reason, my father would spend most of the afternoon with three Sunday papers sitting in the car outside on the street.

If one of his wife's sisters succeeded in cajoling him in at Christmas time with the promise of a turkey sandwich, he would sit on the sofa in the lounge, consume the sandwich, drink the tea, and then off with him again, even on those cold winter days.

'Where are you going?' my mother might ask him in astonishment, seeing him put on his hat.

'I'll go for a walk,' he'd say, and that was the last we might see of him for an hour.

I suppose he was a great walker.

Sometimes I escaped from the chatter in the kitchen, just to sit in the old dining room on the first floor that overlooked the square, and I would see him strolling around or looking into the window of the chipper or the drapery at the other end of the square.

Two hours later he'd appear again at the door of the pub and my mother would rush to him and say, 'Are you ready to go?' and he'd say, 'There's no rush.'

He might as well have brought the standard lamp, the armchair and the drawing room from home with him. It was as if he lived permanently in that solitary space, even when he was not in it.

And I even tried to emulate him, to make for myself a solitary world where I supposed I might come to be like him. And the old dining room upstairs in the pub was a magical room that enchanted me and where I began to feel like him, safely alone.

My aunt inherited the property and after being widowed early in life she fussed around the back rooms with bunches of keys, wondering how she would manage a pub, so she employed a quiet and considerate barman who was as attentive as a good priest with the clientele. He had the temperament of a monk, and he ran the bar on her behalf for decades before her son took over.

I called it an old dining room but everyone else called it the 'parlour' and it was directly above the bar, with an old piano, a nineteenth-century breakfast table and lots of lacework and velvet drapes on the windows. The table was covered with a crocheted shawl. The backs of the rocking chair and other Victorian armchairs were adorned with lace, and place mats for wine glasses were laid out in measured order on the sideboard.

I would lie on the floor as a ten-year-old child and press my ear to the floorboards listening to the male voices in the bar below and imagine the nature of those conversations. The kitchen was full of women chattering and the bar full of men whispering. But up in that room it felt like a monastery, an empty space, a kind of sanctuary.

The pub was always a haven for worried souls. The atmosphere was more of a wellness centre, a temple of meditative quietude. The bus stopped outside the door and people came in for consultations. Everything was whispered as in a confessional.

Clients had their own corners and whispered their troubles to the barman, who bowed his head in silence as he listened. He was bald and wore a white shirt and over that a manly brown leather apron. And he had a very slight limp which gave him further gravitas. Sometimes I imagined snippets of conversation. I imagined people confessing to things they should not have done and spilling out secrets of enormous proportion on the counter.

It surprised me that any soul who had earlier confessed his sins to some priest up the road in a confession box should now come here to drink a pint on a Saturday night and then share his real emotions or confusion with a barman or perhaps some other stranger at the bar. Even at ten years of age I could see that the public house might be a great resource. A place of refuge beyond the imagination of the holy fathers in the clergy.

I was hardly six years old when I first set foot in that lovely Victorian world, and I returned there with my mother regularly through my teenage years, on Sundays. And always in search of that space my father seemed to have found on his solitary walks, where he was content with just his own company.

And the furniture in that room stood outside time. The dining table, the sideboard, the upright piano and the rocking chair, the chaise longue and the sofa; they floated in some timeless reality and heightened for me the notion that time was the grand delusion, and that something else remained forever.

It allowed me to consider reality as fragile. Everything in the room was from a previous century, so it created a disconnect with time: Georgian furniture as fragments of eternity, the debris of history and detritus of the past; artefacts enduring in the wake of an era that had already passed.

Of course I was in my late teens by then, my father old and feeble and no longer able to travel. Old Auntie Nellie was gone to her rest in the local graveyard, as was Auntie Molly and Uncle Bill. But Bernadette was still there, and her son, a charming young star of the local GAA, had taken over the bar. I drove my mother on those few occasions and still liked to take a peek upstairs to see if the upper room was actually still there. Marooned in its own timeless realm.

That was a space where I found refuge. Where I could live outside time, sitting on a Victorian rocking chair and beginning to know my own life as memory.

Such was the melancholy that crept in on me as I finished my Leaving Certificate. No wonder that I was thinking about heading for a seminary to try on the clothes and costumes of a priestly caste and find a role in life whereby I could abandon the world and be consumed by what ancient mystics would call 'the fire of solitude'.

But even still my father's ghost looks in the window, although less frequently now. During winter he is always there on the other side of the glass, standing gaunt in the other world with books by Primo Levi under his arm, inviting me to join him, as he waits beneath the trees in my garden, with the severity of Samuel Beckett.

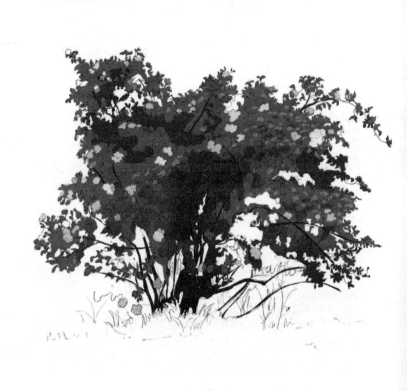

A Light on the Mountain, a Fire in the Stove

For me fire was always an image of solitude. Loneliness had nothing to recommend it, but solitude was a burning flame. It was the presence in the burning bush, the thing that cleansed the soul and that tested gold in the furnace.

Flames contained the merciless wrath of God in my religion books but in reality the flickering flame in the stove carried the lightness of God that extended into the bar and filled the customers with life. Flames in my religion books appeared above the heads of the apostles at Pentecost. It was the moment they found courage and eloquence. And many were the nights when some old farmer waxed effusively in the bar and another customer would comment that he was 'on fire'.

It was especially when I tried to embrace the world in public houses that I noticed how important the flames were. The stove was a mighty allure. The open fire or the pot-bellied stove in any hotel or lounge was the thing I clung to rather than the drink.

It was like the candle in a sanctuary, a living flame signifying safety and welcome. I saw it as a symbol of sacral life beneath the surface of ordinary things. No matter how desperate the faces were, or how tortured their souls were, in public houses at the end of the world where alcoholics clung to the counter like it might be a life raft, and hugged each other in shared despair, yet they saw hope always in the symbol of a fire in the stove. The pub was always where stories grew wilder and songs more tender were sung, and imaginations danced like the flames in the mouth of a furnace.

There was a stove in the Glan Bar, where I took refuge in my twenties, and in Costello's in Skehana, where I took refuge in my thirties, surviving on a bicycle and on oven-cooked pearl rice that I ate alone in a rented bungalow not far from the pub.

And even when I returned to Cavan at one stage as an ordained priest, just five years after my father's death, I found refuge in a bar on Main Street behind the grocery shop, where the stove was always lit.

I had been appointed as a teacher to St Patrick's College in Cavan town and often met folks who would still remark on his passing, recalling how jovial he was at parties in amateur dramatic circles decades earlier. It was like hearing about a stranger. And by then I had my own playacting to do, both in the Christian ministry and as a member of the Hacklers Amateur Drama Group, many of whom frequented that bar.

The bar had a day licence and closed at 6 p.m. each evening. It allowed poets, amateur-dramatic clowns and bored teachers to shorten the day and reach the climax of closing time long before night. The frenzy of last orders occurred at around 5.45 p.m. each evening, which suited clients who were obliged by the constraints of married life to go home for their tea.

But it was always comforting to watch the proprietor coming out into the customer area with a bucket of coal and a shovel to refill the fat metal belly. It was an assurance that we weren't yet at the closing moment, for he would never put coal on the fire after five o'clock.

We lived on borrowed time all afternoon, some only indulging in Paris buns and pots of tea, while the more artistic types smoked dope, and sad civil servants drank with a kind of quiet anguish.

Because in those days everything was permissible so long as you never gave it a name. And there were gay bars and bars where the smell of marijuana would knock a delicate cat unconscious in every town in the country. There were bars where guards drank minerals and sat in the corner dressed in Dunnes Stores jumpers and trousers creased like razor blades as if nobody knew they were guards.

But the great difference between those establishments and the wine bars or coffee shops of today is that those public houses were spaces which reverberated with masculinity; at worst toxic and at best deeply melancholic.

My father's life was a long winter and a late spring. It wasn't an easy journey from the cottage in Donnybrook where he was reared in poverty to the swanky semi-detached house in Cavan where he ended up in the shelter of his beloved.

And that's another aspect of his life that was and remains hidden to me. Whatever the nature of his attachment to my mother, it is shrouded in time and I will never know if he did bring joy to her, and if not, then why not. Even at those Christmas moments in the pub in Castlepollard, my aunts Bernadette and Molly would sing a few lines of an old song, but my mother never joined in.

The secret may have been her feet. I think we all have some secret joy that we cherish and yet try to hide. For her it may have been dancing. She was proud of her dancing as a child. She went to dances in the town hall in Cavan as a young woman, only for the pleasure of dancing with partners that were also at the top of their game. She was noticed by my father, who shared lodgings with a man renowned for the lightness of his feet, and she may have presumed that the lightness was contagious and that by sharing digs with a dancer my father too would possess a pair of shoes to dazzle the town hall. She was wrong but by then it was too late. She was married.

She squeezed her exuberance for life out through her toes for years afterwards at dances or golf-club functions and she spent Sunday afternoons watching Fred Astaire on the television.

Perhaps she still dances in some ballroom of bliss or whatever heavenly realm she was dissolved into.

I often hear people talking about the past as if it was a brutal, loveless place. As if the present is more civilised and as if all the chaste bachelors in Leitrim's glens remained alone because of some terrible damage done in their childhood.

Yet I keep meeting old people, married and single, whose childhood was full of innocence, whose courting was full of tenderness and whose homes were full of love; widows and widowers who still have a spring in their step, or single men who sit contentedly by the fire and talk to the dog.

An undertaker once told me that he was called on to remove a corpse from a bed in a country house. As he lifted the remains from the sheets he could see two distinct hollows in the mattress, where the deceased and his wife had slept side by side for many decades. On the day of the funeral the wife collapsed and died in the graveyard, the bond of love between them unbroken, even in death. So it may have been with my parents.

But the point about human life is that each one of us carries the anxiety of not knowing quite what our parents were like. We search for them in the debris of time, and we find our fathers as an enduring presence inside us. I expected to find my father somewhere, or anywhere, in public houses or on empty streets, even though he had already died. But nonetheless I searched for him in every silence.

And if wholeness is to be found in the balance of male and female, then the decisive night for me came in late July of 1976 when I found myself at a well in the Cuilcagh mountains with the woman of my dreams.

It was she who led me there, and the summer shrubbery of the fields and rolling hills resounded with feminine tenderness. But it was the moon that felt oddly male in that moment. Which surprised me. The pallid blank face conjured up my father's presence instantly, perhaps because the white moon reminded me of his remains, interred just hours earlier.

And the reflection of the moon in the water astonished me. As if some part of him were inside me. I carried him as a mirror carries a greater reality. He was the moon on the surface of a pool. He was a light in the dark, a guiding compass and a witness to all my longing. And I was water. It's why I said I loved him from the day he died. Even though it was misguided of me to think that any fragment of his presence remained in the universe.

My father was gone. That is all there is to it. And yet I was opening this longing for him and this love for him that would afflict me for years.

From that moment I began to carry inside me the dead thing that we call the father-god, like he did in his own time, and men in their thousands, enclosed in silent rooms, private refuge spaces, lonely fields and mountain cottages, or in prison cells, hospital rooms or detention centres do.

I was twenty-two when he died and felt the tug

of the ephemeral moon shimmering on the surface of water and thought that I had found him at last, and that I loved him. All in one day I had buried him, taken refuge in the pub and ended up in the middle of the night at the edge of a well.

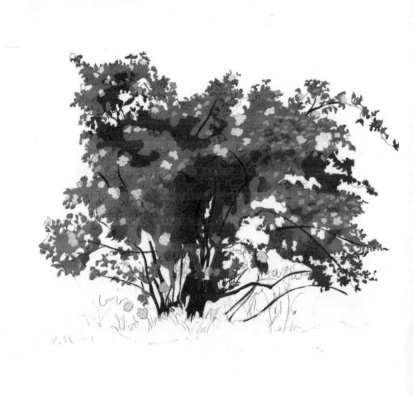

Keep Calm at the Airport

It must have been the water in the airport triggered me. Dublin airport offers bottles of water to passengers by way of honesty boxes scattered around the boarding areas, whereby intending passengers can speedily pick up a bottle and drop two euros in the allotted box without being delayed at a checkout. I took a bottle from the crate, put a two-euro coin in the slot and thought how like a candelabra in a church it was. Just like I'd put my money into the slot before lighting a candle, so I dropped the money in the box beside the crate and took the water. But nesting in this transaction I sensed the remnants of something religious, which is probably why I began thinking of holy wells.

There are always disconnected ruminations that flood my mind when I'm idling the time before a boarding gate in Dublin Airport. And the more I get irritated by the squashed panic of the airport, the more I go inside and dream.

One thing I resent about travelling on planes is the aggression of security staff shouting at the queue about discarding their belts and shoes and getting laptops out of rucksacks. I'm emotionally exhausted by the time I get through security; my trousers are falling down and I'm constantly in danger of forgetting a phone or watch or leaving it in the tray after it has gone through the screening machine.

And another thing that frustrates me is the way people queue for the flight at the boarding gate. They rush to be at the front while the staff checks passports and boarding cards, and then if I am drawn into this collective panic, we all end up in the stairwell for twenty minutes still waiting for staff to vacuum and clean the plane on the apron before we can board and I'm standing there in agony regretting that I drank the water and that I forgot to go to the bathroom.

So, I keep calm by reflecting on the meaning of life, and since I was going to Spain to walk the

Camino I couldn't resist falling into such reveries about various holy wells and watering holes. Places of refuge and comfort. Sanctuaries. Wells. And all the lovely open fires in long-ago bars and lounges, and not least among them the cosy little camp in Glangevlin called the Glan Bar.

But it's a short flight to Santiago, and in the arrivals lounge a man with my name written on a card was waiting with a Mercedes taxi at the door. I took a dash to the bathroom and stood at the urinal giving thanks to God for having allowed the tour company to organise everything for me including taxis; two hours later I checked into my first hotel to begin the pilgrimage from the town of Sarria.

All I had in my yellow backpack was the jacket of a suit, a few changes of underwear, a light rain-proof anorak, my passport, and socks. And a large purse with medicines, tablets and vitamin supplements.

The following morning I ate slices of cold ham, cheese and a hard-boiled egg in the breakfast area of the hotel and headed off across a small river by way of a footbridge and along the suburbs of

Sarria, following the bright yellow arrows on blue backgrounds which were placed like tiles in various walls and at corners of streets to lead the pilgrims into the countryside and just a little closer to Santiago.

It was 7.30 a.m. The temperature was in the high teens. Soon it would reach the low thirties. I needed to reach my destination by midday before it got too hot.

I wished for rain, but it was Thursday and no rain was promised until the end of the following week, which seemed like a very long way off.

And as I walked through streets on the edge of town I passed the scallop shell again and again. A shell, which I remembered from my childhood as a symbol for a brand of petrol, had become the great symbol of the Camino, because in centuries gone by the actual scallop shells were used as directional markers for pilgrims. Now it manifests everywhere, not just as tiles in walls, or on shop-fronts, but as actual shells that dangle from the pilgrims' backpacks.

Maybe I was expecting to see pilgrims with rosary beads dangling around their necks, or images of St James sewn into backpacks, but the odd thing about my Camino is that it didn't feel religious and the pilgrims walking behind and before me, in their hundreds, dining in the same restaurants and coffee houses along the way, never looked like they had the slightest interest in religion. The young lived on their smartphones, and the middle-aged and elderly kept their chins up and looked like any pack of healthy hikers.

I wasn't saying any prayers, and I saw no other pilgrim on their knees at any point. Quite the opposite; here was a great horde of young Europeans, being young and sizzling with affection for each other and discussing the merits of a vegan diet and laughing in the evenings over their wine and pasta. Clearly this was a walking holiday.

The only thing about the hordes of young people in T-shirts and shorts that I resented was how supple their bodies were and how briskly they could pass me on the pathways with enormous rucksacks on their backs and me breathless, sweating, barely able to get up the hills, with only a little yellow rucksack full of blood pressure tablets.

It's well for them, I thought. And then I went inside again. Allowing the endless rhythm of walking to work on my mind until I was back again in the cave of the heart, where I clutched icons and imaginal constructs and dreamed deeply of my father.

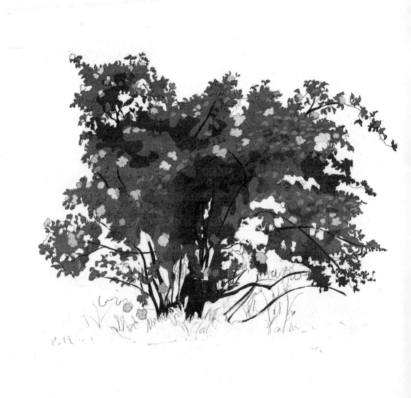

Never Forget

Glangevlin, that mountain parish in west Cavan, exists also for me in the remembrance of it. The geographic location, the space in time that corresponds to what is on the map, was never the real Glangevlin for me. My mind reshaped it as a memory; something I now cherish in the eternal present.

So, I might have been walking from Sarria to Morgade on the first day, or Morgade to Portomarin on the second day, and so on as far as Santiago, but on the inside I never quite left Glangevlin or the pool of water where the moon floated like dead bones.

On the map Glangevlin is a small parish in the Cuilcagh mountains where the river Shannon rises. The river source or 'pot' is a large pool, a deep and mysterious well celebrated in ancient folktales and hidden by hawthorns on the slope of the mountain. The parish was once an independent tribal community of clans dominated by McGoverns, who governed themselves in small things for centuries, speaking Irish well up to the end of the nineteenth century and holding tight to their sheep and mountain farms through the twentieth despite the impoverishment that came with the new Free State and the lure of London and Chicago. But in the end Glangevlin fell into a state of quiet resignation that typifies many sparsely populated corners of rural Ireland as they watch the sitka trees grow up and darken all their lovely childhood playgrounds.

I remember old men talking in the bar about the fun they'd had in years gone by. I was still a boy in 1973 but those old men still relished the antics of their youth and got joy from the simple act of remembering.

Just after the Second World War, Cavan town hosted a military tattoo to celebrate the life and times of Owen Roe O'Neill. General O'Neill was an Irish warrior and chief who had fought with the French and gathered a great army of resistance across Ulster in the seventeenth century to fight the English, winning victory at the Battle of Benburb. It was the last great victory of a native Gaelic army against the English, although the advantage was subsequently wasted by mismanagement, and the great General O'Neill died in 1649 at the hands of his enemies.

In the mid-twentieth century Ireland was enduring a splendid isolation after a botched War of Independence which resulted in the devastating partition of the island. In 1949 Europe was in flux and yet another deluge of change was sweeping across the continent, but the town of Cavan was celebrating not the end of war or the death of Hitler but the three-hundredth anniversary of General O'Neill's death and other facets of Ireland's tribal argument with the English.

The festivities in Cavan town opened with a day of parades and speeches, and in attendance were some young blades from Glangevlin – teenage boys drinking stout and smoking until their eyes came out on sticks.

They returned that night to the peaceful hills of their home place, unsatisfied by the dull and

tedious ceremonies in the town. For further enter-
tainment they decided to turn the peaceful hills
of Glan into a carnival of anarchy and confusion.

This they did by calling at houses, shouting in
windows, all sorts of strange tales of woe, in voices
of familiar neighbours.

'Mrs so-and-so is having her baby, come quick!'

'Tommy so-and-so is taken ill, he'll not last till
morning!'

'The big brown cow is stuck in the ditch, you
better come out!'

A different tale at every house. All in the mask
of another person's voice. And at sufficient houses
to create a busy stir on the roads.

Soon people and lamps were moving over the
hills in all directions. They passed each other in
the black night, suspicious and mystified at first.

'Hi, where are you going?'

'I know where I'm going, but where the hell are
you going?'

When they finally realised what was afoot, they
mobilised into search parties to find the young
rascals. The boys lay low in the ditches while grey-
haired men stalked the roadways, in their shirts

and tails. The young blades would laugh tears for weeks, remembering all that manhood swinging in the wind.

Of course, they knew also that if they were caught, they would pay dearly. The fur would fly.

An edgy suspicion infected social life for weeks. Old men stared at young men in long shafts of silence. The whetstone made a slow, disturbed sound on the billhook.

But in the end, no one was ever found out, and the secret of who turned the peaceful hills of Glan into such turmoil that night was never revealed. A song was made about the incident which ridiculed the victims, and its rendition at wedding or in public house was often followed by heated debate.

Those were the kinds of stories I heard during my first winter in Glangevlin, as I taught school by day and socialised in the Glan Bar by night. Older men who remembered those events of long ago would relate them with relish and fun. My father was forty-seven years dead in 2023 but back then his health was in decline and I found comfort listening to the legends of what I saw as heroic and invincible mountain men, because they were so radically different from the fragile father lingering in the faraway drawing room of a semi-detached house in small-town suburbia.

The boys of that night had become the men beside me. I was the boy beside them, wishing I too was a man as robust and abrasive as them.

My own father, a newly appointed accountant in the local county council who had previously worked for Clare County Council, must have been around Cavan in 1949, paying court to his future wife and dreaming about building a house and home in which I was born four years later.

But how different the lives of those Glangevlin mountain farmers were in that long-ago time, I thought. While my father watched the construction of the house where I was reared, the young lads of Glangevlin were tumbling around in the night with the abandon of people who have nothing to build.

By the time I heard such stories in the Glan Bar my father was nursing a sore hip and sitting all day with a tartan rug across his knees, while these old men were still robust and strong from walking the mountain after sheep and cycling their bicycles home from the pub at night. Even in old age my father was about to lose everything, and these old men had nothing to lose.

But it was the fluidity with which the stories rose around the flaming stove in the Glan Bar that excited me. More stories in a single night than in an entire childhood spent in the quiet sobriety of Cavan town.

How could old men be so loquacious? I wondered. Without pain or sentimentality, they could talk like heroes and tell stories until morning. How I wished to be like them. And how magically did their memories create a strange sense of intimacy so that age and time dissolved and we stood in the one eternal present.

The remembrance of things became its own meaning beyond time. And when Rose, the proprietor, occasionally and gently announced closing time and asked the old men had they homes they might think of going to, she was invariably dismissed, with a gentle firmness, as if the notion of time could disrupt the eternal present when one had just one more story to tell and one more glass of whiskey to finish.

Although regarding the identity of those young blades, no one said much back in 1976. 'The old ones are all dead and gone,' they sang, 'the young ones turning grey.'

And even then, the drift of people from the hills of Cuilcagh to the suburbs of New York continued so that those heroes ended their days surrounded by the budding sitka forests that finally swallowed everything. In Glangevlin today the forestry is peppered with little empty shells that once were homesteads. I saw them all as heroic, braving life with vigour, whiskey, a few stories and a song. The contrast with my own father was stark. He was a man I could never imagine risking himself to any outrageous pranks in the middle of the night or livening up some public house by the remembrance of it. He was dull. And worse than that, he was virtuous.

It's funny how the young despise virtue and long to commit acts of boldness and deviance. I sat between the two stools: my father's discreet life as an accountant sitting with his books, and the rugged wilderness that these old heroes inhabited in their youth and sang about in old age. Two versions of masculinity, I suppose. The one being coy and careful, discreet and reflective. The other being as abrasive as a song sung long after closing time.

But the irony is that my father's voice still sings in me many decades after his demise, whereas in rural Ireland the sitka forest triumphed as the English did over General O'Neill; and the wind whistles now through the tumbled walls of those old houses in Glangevlin and even the story of who they were has been forgotten.

One way or another, it was certainly in the Glan Bar that I met my father's ghost at twenty-one years of age, though I didn't know it was my father at the time, and I didn't know who the fragile seventy-one-year-old retired accountant in Cavan was either. Because in physical terms the weak, declining person he had become could not contain the sense of fatherhood I longed for.

So how could I know who I had buried on that day in late July 1976? A dead moon had sunk into the clay of a Cavan graveyard and then surfaced in my heart twelve hours later.

I looked into the eyes of a man twice my age in Glangevlin who had returned from America, who lived with his sheep, who had large hands like chunks of an oak tree and veins like rivers running under the skin, and smoked and drank bottles of Guinness, and he said, 'Let me get you a drink, you've been through a lot.'

That was the hug. That was the tenderness I had been missing. That was my father.

And the lovely sheep were never far away. I could smell them off men's clothes at the bar. I could see them outside my window. I could hear them in the night. I could get frustrated when my old Cortina was blocked by a large flock being herded from their scraggy rush-covered sheltering places in the hills to the dipping units along the main road. And in the pub after a fair in Dowra the lounge swelled with animated conversation and sticks were levelled along the counter and sheep shite on wellingtons offered up a pungent aroma to mix with the whiskey in the air and the milky aftertaste of Guinness.

I was a young hero leaping across the drumlins of Cavan, trying to lure women into my arms with the prospect of driving them to dances in a broken-down car with a wobbly steering wheel. The night was always a destination and there was never any tomorrow, and the watering hole along the road was always the Glan Bar.

Sometimes before a dance, girls gathered in clusters on the soft cushions of the lounge while boyfriends clung to the counter of the bar. The sexes were separated as strictly as at a Taliban wedding, until the final moment when a boy would drain his glass, duck his head below the lintel and go through the low door to the lounge.

'Are you coming?' was all that he muttered gruffly to his girlfriend.

'No,' she might retort, for the amusement of her friends, 'I'm only breathing heavy.'

But nonetheless she went with him, out into the night to the carpark at the back of the bar or across the street to Mrs Dolan's post office shop and she might be moderately satisfied with her boyfriend's sparkling old banger and the furry seat covers, bought at Mullen Mart on the border and an

8-track stereo tape deck stuck into the dashboard, pumping out the music of country singers from Tyrone.

The bar was floored with cement and well suited for wellingtons, but the lounge was carpeted, with dainty lights on the walls above a modern mantelpiece and an open fire that was hot enough to roast the arses off musicians, poets, sheep farmers, singing postmen, teachers and prison officers. Musicians sweated through the armpits of their flower-patterned shirts, and women waiting on their lovely boys kept cool by holding their backs to the walls behind them and staying as far away from the blazing furnace as possible.

Although the women were not without agency. Some were teachers and nurses and cooks in the local prison and barmaids and factory workers in Ballinamore. Some worked closer to home in a small meat-packing factory started by a returned exile from America.

Not that we knew what vacuum-packed meat was before the Yank came to start the factory. The notion of sealing a pair of sirloin steaks or four centre loin chops in plastic with a machine that looked like a photocopier was something we ridiculed behind the Yank's back, at house parties, around the dinner table or at the range in the kitchen of the bar.

When we moved about in the small hours of the night we knew the hills were full of other people moving guns across the border, or men on the run in search of safe houses, and at every crossroads there was the possibility of guards with flashlights and blue luminous signs on the road that said 'Checkpoint', behind which there lurked the diminutive little soldiers of the Irish army.

If we were asked where we were going on our way out the Gap, the mountain pass that linked the isolated parish of Glangevlin to the rest of the world and which we crossed on weekends going to dances in Drumshanbo, we might say that we were heading for New York. Or that we didn't know. Or that we had not decided if we were going to Dublin or Timbuktu.

We were now the smart-alecky young blades. We might not climb on top of the roof to block someone's chimney but at least we gave the guards a hard time. And on the way home if a guard asked where we were going as he gawked into the car as if he were a half-wit, we'd say, 'We're going home, guard. For fuck sake, at this hour of the night where do you think we're going? And maybe you should fuck off home yourself, guard.'

This bollocky attitude was tolerated by the guards because they too were young and regularly appeared in dancehalls around the area on their nights off. They never darkened the door of the pub, but they danced in the same halls and listened to the same music as the local women who sometimes ended up as girlfriends, wives and then mothers to the children of those same officers.

So, the guards took the abuse, but we knew they were okay, because they always won the approval of the women. I often noticed them snooping about the back yard, and occasionally a sergeant would plonk himself at the range in the kitchen of the bar, ostensibly to be sociable but ultimately in the hope of hearing little nuggets of information that might sustain him in his search for terrorists. But I never saw a guard in the bar in those years. The elders at the bar were predominantly celibate farmers, even if some of them were married, whose attachment was to their sheep dogs. Black and white beauties that sat under the chairs, or remained out in the yard, or sometimes in the back of an old man's Ford Anglia.

And all the while the Guinness and beer flowed, not from taps on draught but from enormous pint bottles, until the counter was stacked like a storeroom of empties, and then whiskeys were poured, as luminous as melting amber, and by midnight it flowed without measure.

It's just that there was no courting in the bar. The lounge was the place for mixing the sexes. The quiet misogynistic calm in the bar was like the scent of a bull sleeping in a field. A beast that no one would want to waken.

If there wasn't a major event in the lounge, then the only place with lights on was the bar. It would stay open until late. Young ladies might be at home in the bath or drying their hair and decking their arms and necks with bracelets and necklaces as they waited for men to come collect them around 11 p.m., or even later. Then the cars would head off to dancehalls scattered across three counties with young lads who had spent the evening drinking in the pub. The women would have to wait because they had no choice. The bar was a congress of masculinity, and nobody spoke of anything as tender as love.

When those young lads went off to fetch their girlfriends, the remnant in the bar looked even older, more desperate for another drink and sublimely alone. They had bicycles outside heaped up against the wall of the loft. They had plastic coal bags to pin to their shoulders and protect themselves from the rain on the way home. And a few of us, like me, a school-teacher, or the local priest, or the manager of the vacuum-packing factory that employed three people, would retire to the kitchen for tea and bacon sandwiches before we too drove away separately in our cars. Vesty, a brother to the proprietor and devoted barman, would wander in and out as he collected empty bottles from the bar and stacked them in crates just outside the kitchen door, for the beer trucks to collect on the following morning, and some-times he'd see the scattering of us devouring sandwiches and drinking mugs of tea around the kitchen table, and he'd say, 'I see the high and mighty are gathered again,' as he eyed me and the priest and the Yank and a few others scoffing the sandwiches. But to me I was part of more than the high and mighty. I was in my father's house. I belonged in that kitchen, in that bar, in that mountain parish, more than I had ever felt in the little bedroom in Cavan where I grew up.

In Glan the wilderness was outside the door and when I stretched on the bed at night I could feel the earth below the foundations of the house hold me up, and the willows being battered by the wind outside the window whispered love songs to me.

Surely that must be the power of the father, I thought.

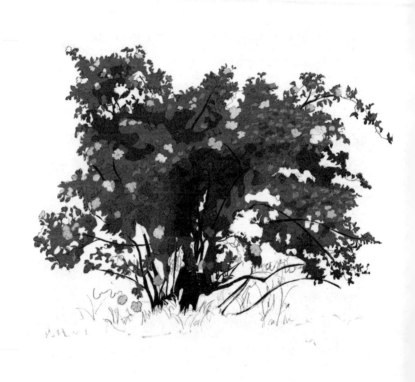

Who Is at the Door?

And in the kitchen of the bar, we neglected no topic that might have been flagged on the television news.

We spoke of wars in Asia and drugs in Dublin, communism in Russia and life in American universities. We spoke of vacuum-packed meat and pirate radio stations.

But we never spoke of the war outside the door, up on the mountain; the existential threat to the state of Northern Ireland, on the edge of which we scratched around and lived our small lives.

Glangevlin was perched in an isolated dip in the mountains, and over the hills on many fronts was Northern Ireland, and over the other hills was Leitrim, a place where senior IRA leaders sometimes appeared on the back of lorries in town squares to thank the people of Leitrim for their prayers and their houses. War was simply too dangerous to speak of.

But we never spoke of love either, because there was no need to. When a man was leaving to pick up a girlfriend nobody bade him goodnight. He would slip away from the bar as heroic as anyone going to war who knows he must never return.

In my early twenties this failure to acknowledge love felt right. And when my father spoke of the grandmother he loved, or my mother down in the kitchen whom he loved, or when he spoke just in general terms about the good weather and the roses blooming in the back garden, he exuded a kind of lightness that I found squeamish. Speaking of love was sentimental. And the lurking presence of Clint Eastwood on the cinema screen seemed more akin to the understated endurance that was required when one of the boys got distracted by a girlfriend and betrayed the company of men at the bar.

Because every departure from the bar was a betrayal if it was for the sake of fussing over some girl. Such restraint in the matter of love and romance was oddly at variance with my father's gushing enthusiasm for the world. I thought him sentimental. I thought the boys in the bar were real men. And I had no idea back then of how male insecurity shelters itself in a mask of true grit and how vulnerability is actually the true face of love.

The men's ability to blank out a particular topic or person was never more evident than when a stranger would arrive. A traveller from God-knows-where would darken the door, lean against the counter for a few whiskeys and then vanish without a farewell. Nobody gave him a name. Nobody gave a damn who he was. In the space of a tune on the fiddle or the chorus of a song he was forgotten. Nobody remembered him even being there.

I thought of us as philosophers; we could discuss a metaphysical idea without relating it to politics. We could discuss politics without relating it to the personal. And we never discussed the personal. We were akin to peoples in the snowy mountains of Tibet: stoic philosophers minding sheep and with the ability to avoid certain subjects, speak with discretion and embrace the terrible emptiness of life at the end of each night. Mountain people who looked suffering in the eye and enjoyed an Asian perception regarding the philosophical notion of emptiness or the non-existence of the self.

It was most evident when someone died. When the burial was over. The grieving was ended, and the wake had finished. The death would be alluded to in the bar with the most minimal of handshakes. And as often as not it would be shrugged off.

'Ah sure, he is better off where he is now. Won't we all end in the same ground.'

But in the quiet pubs of Ireland this stoicism hid something different from the serenity of Asian philosophers.

The silence of the Asian monk stems from the fact that everything has been said. The reticence of the old men around me stemmed from the fact that nothing could be said.

Behind the silence of a monastery there nestles the idea that even the self does not exist. But in the Glan Bar, silence was a mask that hid a self which everyone was ashamed of.

Failed relationships, broken friendships, family misunderstandings, family feuds and suicides and grief; all reflected on the men that fled to the public house for emotional belonging. They felt like failures. And everyone carried with them what they were ashamed of.

But when there was no death to dwell on, people talked freely, endlessly and with more and more passion and fury as the night wore on. A banter which also masked the private self, or the fragrance of inner pain. Irish men at the time played language games with each other like the Russian game of masquerade; it was a fluency about everything but the truth.

My father never went to public houses. Maybe because he was too old, or because he was an accountant and didn't want to mix with riff-raff, or maybe he had frequented enough pubs when he was young and felt that a good husband is someone who sits at home every evening, like the monarch of his household, at the top of the table tapping the shell of his boiled egg with a teaspoon.

I asked him once why he read only books about philosophy and history, and not novels, like the ones that were on my Leaving Certificate course. He said that at a certain age you don't need novels anymore. 'It's as if everything has been said.'

In the Glan Bar I saw a man from God-knows-where raise the latch many times on the back door in his long coat and slip to the counter for his libation in whispered tones, and I often imagined it might have been my father in that coat. I'd look at the back of his head and wonder why I was feeling the same anxiety I had when I saw the back of my father's head.

And I hadn't a clue that it was simply because my father too was a stranger, unidentified and unquestioned.

After the funeral when I found myself at the end of the day in the bar, his absence was sealed. I would never speak with him again. And among the lonely men I began to cry because I realised that I had lost something profound in the moment of his death and I had not appreciated it when it was available to me.

It was a hot night. A warm summer night in July. But I was there on other nights too, in winter. And in winter snow fell with confidence from early January to the middle of February. People came in the door from a blizzard in the yard and returned into the middle of the same blizzard hours later. We were all wet, perished and equal. All together in a haze of alcohol and blissful ignorance.

The difference, just like philosophers again, was that we knew we were ignorant. We knew how little we knew, and we knew where it all ended, no matter what your erudition, wealth or love affairs.

Some men were rich from working on the buildings in London. And others hadn't even the price of a drink. And they used to say in those years that a man could go to New York and change his life around in five years. They spoke of the building sites in London or Manchester as if they were battlefields where spoils could be won that might transform an entire life and endow a man with kingship. A man might end up coming home to Glan someday in a Mercedes. And some of those too were among us, especially in summertime. And no better place for those kings to be than in the Glan Bar, the big blue Merc sitting outside the door, as they bought everyone a drink to assure us that life was sweet and easy.

In a sense they had all the riches of the world that passed my father by as he clung to a small non-incremental pension for the last years of his life.

The summer brought many such visitors who made us feel good and inflated, but when they left their absence punctured our illusions. The men around me were diminished.

On bleak winter evenings we were all touched by a hint of self-loathing; we were the dregs left behind that were not quite able for America or London.

I've always found that men have a powerful tendency to indulge despair. It's as if the only intimacy possible is the necessary intimacy of death and mortality. *We are all the same when we're in the ground* is a powerful equalising and consoling idea in any bar. Pain and hopelessness can forge a bond of bleak solidarity. Despair was open, shared and comforting. And it comforted me too.

That we would all end up in the same dead silence that covered the earth. In the same snow that covered the remains of dead monks in Tibet or the same wind that blew through the bare bones of dead horses in the deserts of Timbuktu.

And it's no exaggeration to say that people in Tibet or Timbuktu or Glangevlin all have a common wisdom about the contingencies of life, the passing of time and the silence that falls eventually on us all.

They were pilgrims, living in a medieval world despite the rumours of something called modernity. The men around me knew this. They knew themselves in all their poverty. They were not unconscious. But like all indigenous people they had no hope in the face of modernity.

My father, on the other hand, was never done bemoaning his desperate situation as a child, selling newspapers on the street, unable to attend secondary school, packing boxes in a large city store, and then recounting with joy and triumph his own transformation and achievements in finally securing a good profession, a wife and children, all packed into the perfect semi-detached house with a garden to the front and rear.

It's as if his life was a success and I as a youth was in no frame of mind to rejoice in that.

Especially since his health was in such decline that it certainly didn't look like a success to me. His children away at university. His wife off in the golf club playing nine holes with her friends from the Irish Countrywomen's Association. It seemed perverse that he expressed contentment in his armchair. And the last thing I wanted to see before me was his frail little body. Far more acceptable were the despondent farmers lugging themselves to the bar and leaning their huge frames over the counter as they sipped strong liquor and spoke of the mountains they wrestled with. They were not in declining health like my father. They were not sitting satisfied in their drawing rooms reading books by dead monks. They were enduring rough weather, slaughtered by poverty and loneliness, but they were singing. They were men. And my father ought to be among them. Perhaps he was, and perhaps the old man in the drawing room was not to be reckoned with.

I was an exception in their world. I had been to college. I was a teacher and they attributed to me the title of master.

'Forgive me, master,' they would say, 'but I am an unlettered person.'

With all their soft affection for donkeys, motor-bikes and sheepdogs, their astonishing mix of brutish courage in the face of foddering animals high on the mountains in winter storms, their deference and reverence for education and their innate Buddhist passivity about the nature of suffering and the certainty of death, how could I resist them?

They weren't my father. And then in some nebulous way they became my father. Like a murmuration of starlings, I could see the form of something beautiful in them.

Unschooled they may have been, and inartic-ulate about their emotions, but not lacking compassion. In fact, during summertime when the bar was occasionally peppered with men who had spent decades on oil rigs, crossed the deserts of Africa in trucks or raised families in Queens or Brooklyn before returning home to die like old salmon, someone would sing a song about emigration and no one would be ashamed to say that there was a tear in their eye. That was as close as it got to intimacy in a world of true grit.

Rose McGovern, the owner and chief bar person, allowed the drinking to go on just thirty minutes longer than the legal time, and occasionally would invite a few men left standing to the kitchen where she could sober them up with bacon sandwiches, before organising lifts home for old bachelors who had abandoned their bicycles at the wall outside Peg Dolan's post office shop hours earlier when they were collecting their dole money. And in the kitchen fathers who had given their children lifts to dancehalls would sup mugs of tea and wait until two in the morning when they would drive again all the way back to the ballroom to collect their children and often the neighbours' children and drive them home. The kitchen was a sacred space, an inner sanctum; it sobered us at the end of the night, replenished us with libations as water sustains a dry, weary land. As water sustains cattle in fields and sheep on the mountain.

But for the elders the end of the night was a bicycle lamp, a last cigarette at the gable, a plastic sack around an old man's shoulders staggering off into the sleet. The end of the night brought silence. The back yard filled with whispers and forgiveness, where nothing ever spoken was repeated in daylight. We went out to the yard and across to a shed a final time, where the cement floor and the aluminium trough sufficed for two or four men to urinate together in silence. We pissed with pleasure, and grateful for the stars above us in the yard.

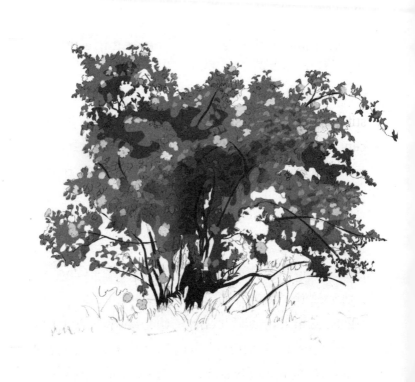

My Heart's Compass

I wore a suit on the Camino. I bought it in a charity shop in Castlerea. A double-breasted jacket with wide peak lapels and the Jones New York label stitched onto the inside breast pocket. It was 85 per cent wool and 15 per cent silk which gave the brown colour a sort of sheen, more like black. At first I thought it was a ladies' suit, because it was on the women's rack, but I quickly googled 'Jones New York men's suit' and discovered that I was safe enough purchasing it for fifteen euro. As I began the Camino I placed the brown jacket inside my little yellow rucksack and braved it out on the road wearing the long trousers. I couldn't handle the idea of short trousers. Admittedly some pilgrims on the pathway seemed to brazen their bare old legs triumphantly; their ankle-high boots and mountain walking socks sometimes seemed completely unnecessary on a warm day. And they would look askance at me in long silky trousers. But the silk was keeping me cool. The length of trouser was protecting me from nasty little bug bites. On the first day I wore Hoka shoes, which didn't turn out to be very successful for the long march, but after that I wore sandals so my feet were cool in the evenings.

Some pilgrims carried walking sticks that looked like they were cut from the branches of a tree that morning. And others had metal walking sticks with rubber handles. There were all forms of straw hats, baseball caps and wide-brimmed cowboy hats. One fellow even wore a woollen hat which I suspect did nothing good for his health in the heat of a summer's day. And nearly everyone carried a white scallop shell, with a cross like a sword on the outer side.

I think it's probably important to have a uniform on pilgrimage – a set of clothes with meaning. When you put such clothes on in the morning they resemble the vestments of a monk, a habit or robe which is purposed for a certain task.

The task is to walk, and the walking is easier if you dress for it. And when the day is done, the clothes are washed in the shower or bath and dried on the radiator or on some balcony chair as if the work was a prayer to complete the day.

Only when the clothes are thus refreshed does the pilgrim feel that the rituals of the day have been completed and everything is ready to repeat the same cycle on the morrow.

I liked my brown suit, not just because the silk ran through it or because it distanced me from all other pilgrims, but because the brown felt like the right colour; like a gesture of solidarity with ancient monks who would have walked in brown habits on the same path. But the real value of such uniforms is that they divest the pilgrim of their normal mundane self. As pilgrims in Mecca robe in white and discard their mundane life, so everyone who sets out on a pilgrimage to some awakening must let go of their old self, and boots, walking socks, shorts and rucksacks all facilitate that ancient rite of passage, albeit in modern garments.

But make no doubt that after breakfast in every *albergue* and hotel along the route, while the big cases of luggage are being gathered in the foyer for a taxi to transport to the next hotel, the day's destination, all the souls in boots and rucksacks have left their old selves behind and are heading out the door to face a new encounter with whatever mentor deity makes them tick, as they walk the walk in their holy robes.

Personally, I didn't feel I had a mentor deity on the pilgrimage. But I would wrap myself each morning in the robes I had designated for the journey and head into the sun – or on some mornings under a soft mist – to walk another day in the heat. And before long my father would rise as a presence around me and I began to pay him attention. My dead father, old dry bones in the grave, or a mythic ghost buried in memories of life in Glangevlin, or perhaps ultimately just an all-enveloping presence; the mentor deity that towered above me like the sun in the day and the moon at night, and my heart's compass.

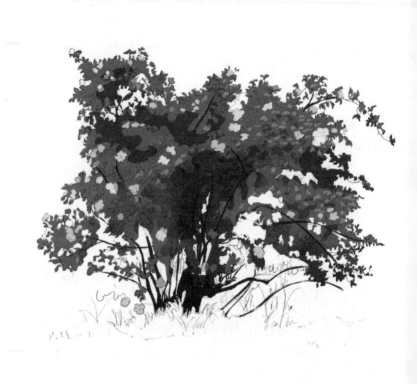

The Moon in the Well

My father died in 1976 after a long withering in a Cavan hospital. I had been teaching in Loughan House since 1974, an open prison near Blacklion, a small village on the border with Northern Ireland, and commuting daily from the mountain parish of Glangevlin, spending my time with mountain folk and falling in love with every young woman who gave me the slightest attention while at the same time being minded by the mothers of the parish and charmed by the raw masculinity of unlettered men who scraped a livelihood coming and going from the hillsides, foddering scrawny cattle and dipping ragged sheep.

My father bade me farewell one Saturday afternoon, reaching his white arm above the blanket and waving at me before pointing his finger into the sky and making a joke about there being an angel hovering above us. It was my final visit to the hospital before he passed.

I wrote in later years of my lifelong love for my wife and partner, and my grief at losing my mother, and my melancholy, despondency and other troubles with health.

But my father's ghost endured as a shadow, a simple longing in me that surfaced sometimes under a full moon in lonely places, like woodlands where holy wells were hidden. Fragments of him lingered in the darkness beneath the May bush. Or on the surface of a pool that held the moonlight.

The day my father died I was in Glangevlin having my hair cut by a young woman when the message came by telephone from the matron in Cavan hospital, Sister Mercy, telling me of his death. I returned to the hair-cutting in the kitchen, but I longed to hold someone. Anyone. Maybe the nun at the other end of the phone, or even the young woman who was clipping my hair in tufts from the back of my head. But I couldn't release myself from the sense of emptiness inside.

It wasn't a gush of emotion for some daddy I loved. It was more a numb awakening. The nun spoke of it being a beautiful moment.

He ate a scone and took some tea from the flask my mother brought to the hospital bed each afternoon. He touched her hand and muttered an often-used cliché when she turned up with food. 'You're very good.'

She thought he looked a bit pale as he closed his eyes, and she went for the nurse. But as the nun said, he was already gone.

My last encounter with him in the hospital, when he waved at me and joked about angels, had changed my memory of his fading body, his white paper-thin skin, into something heroic; an icon of someone surrendering to the angels. His death described by the nun now seemed like a triumph.

Surrendering didn't sound like defeat. The nun did not follow the modern palliative-care line of holding ruthlessly to reality. She did not say, 'He is dead.'

Instead, she held to the more mythic and flowery language of earlier times.

'Your daddy is gone to heaven,' she declared.

Instantly I recalled the moment of humour in his dying that was my last encounter with him. But the ornate language of myth that the nun used gave me permission to love him from that moment onwards in ways I didn't understand.

I loved him fiercely now that he was 'in heaven'. The phrase gave a sense of completion to his life, a satisfying finish to the arc of his story. But it wasn't personal. I felt no great intimacy with him; he had finished his journey elegantly, that's all; and a sense of space inside me was opened up where the heart should be and I felt I was meeting my father there for the first time.

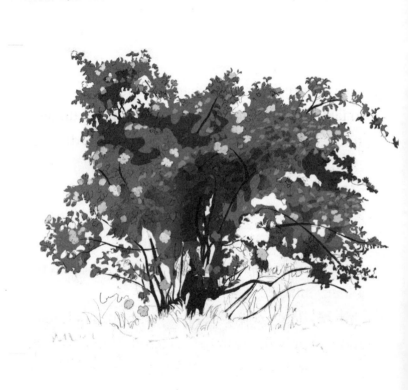

Small Moments Young Men Run a Mile From

Long before his passing I had been devoting myself to father figures with more emotion than I understood. Because when a father is about to die the child must find another parent.

I remember on St Patrick's Day of that year I had a flask of whiskey in my hip pocket and a commission to drive a musician to Blacklion. He was an elderly man who lived alone at the end of a long untarred laneway.

In his damp cottage he lived with a cat, a fiddle and a supply of cigarettes which he clung to like they were his oxygen supply, though his lungs were destroyed.

'I can't breathe at night,' he joked, as I stepped into the dark kitchen.

I was a member of the Cloonclare Drama Group

when I lived in Glangevlin. It was an amateur drama group in Glenfarne, about fifteen miles away, and sometimes after a production of some John B. Keane play I'd end up drinking in the Bush Bar in Blacklion with other members of the cast. I might leave at two in the morning or even later, knowing that my trajectory home was up the hills into Glangevlin where there was little danger of meeting traffic and which I considered a safe enough drive if I managed to keep between the ditches.

Sometimes I'd pass by the laneway to his house, which stood on a remote hill, and I might see lights on in the downstairs kitchen. If I did so, I would park at the gate and walk up the lane, venturing in to find him often on a hard seat with a blanket around his shoulders as he stared at empty ashes in the fire grate. On the surface it may have appeared like I had a hunger for drink when I lifted the latch on his back door. But what I couldn't admit was that he held some strength in his silence that I longed for. He was the wise man in the back of the cave that I couldn't stay away from.

I drove him to the hospital on one occasion, dropping him at the main entrance and then waiting for him in the carpark. When he returned to the car after his consultation he said, 'They told me that if the chest doesn't clear up soon they'll drain it. It makes me sound like a field.'

I laughed because I was familiar with the sound of his lungs, and the way he always struggled much like a drowning man and then made jokes about his condition. Sometimes when I took him to pubs in far-off towns I'd encourage the barman to put on the television because it masked the wheeze when he struggled to get air. Otherwise customers would listen like stunned rabbits to his chest as if he were about to keel over. But it didn't stop him drinking. And it didn't stop me accepting his affliction as normal.

After he discovered inhalers he was as right as rain for about two mornings out of three. Or so he said. But if he took a notion to go looking for sheep on a cold morning I'd find him struggling on the sofa in the afternoon 'like a salmon on dry land'.

On St Patrick's Day he was dressed like an

undertaker, in a black suit with a brown shirt and a psychedelic tie. The birds were singing and a few crocuses were up under the hedge outside his door. His fiddle was lying on a kitchen chair.

'I have an appointment with a flute player from Kiltyclogher,' he said, and he was hugely excited. 'He said he'd meet us in the Black,' he explained as he sat into my new orange Ford Escort. By 'the Black' he meant the town of Blacklion. He could barely breathe.

'Are you okay?'

'I'm fine,' he replied, 'but this fella is an all-Ireland champion. I must meet him.'

We started in the Bush Bar. Vincent McGovern, known as 'Vincie the Bush', was behind the counter, a good-looking man some years my senior. He put up two pints on the counter, eyed the fiddle and refused to take money. In those days musical instruments were a useful means of procuring drink. Musicians would play all day and think themselves lucky if they got a free pint. It never occurred to them that they should be paid for entertaining the other customers.

We put the pints away, as they say, and sat watching the clock, though his friend never arrived. After a while we went down the street to Frank Eddie's, or Frank Maguire's according to the sign above the door. But his friend didn't appear there either and so we headed past the Irish army checkpoint and across the street to Dolan's, a small grocery shop with a day licence to sell alcohol, but that was closed for the day and my friend stood outside, wheezing in confusion.

'He bit-a-be in Belcoo,' he said, which, translated from Hiberno-English, might mean 'he better be in Belcoo' or 'He probably is in Belcoo' – a village across the bridge in Northern Ireland. And only the bridge separated the two main streets.

So off we went, walking across the bridge into Fermanagh, where the IRA used to fire mortars at the army barracks after dark and where three part-time policemen were blown to smithereens under a big oak tree by the same republicans. My eye always caught the tree, and I would think how beautiful it was and how sad that men would plant explosives beneath it just to kill their neighbours.

We passed the old schoolhouse, and a SPAR

shop, and beyond that we arrived at Leo's tavern, a dainty little lounge with a plush carpet which was uncommonly posh in those days. We sat bewildered on high stools, and another customer remarked that we looked like men on a mission.

'We're heading home,' the musician said abruptly. I could see he was devastated. His shrivelled sprig of shamrock hung from a pin on his lapel like an exhausted ballerina and his violin lay silent on the plush red couch behind us.

I spoke to a stranger at the bar about the weather and parades, and how there wasn't as much fun as long ago, but the musician neither drank his pint nor spoke. I was draining my glass when he whispered once again in my ear.

'Take me home.'

It was an order. And I did.

He left the car without farewell, and hurried up his fuchsia lane, and I waited as he scrambled with the key and vanished into the dark. I knew that if I waited long enough I might have heard him play within – 'The Dark-Haired Girl', 'The Battering Ram' or 'My Darling Is Sleeping', which were his favourites. In fact I could have gone in and shared a flask of whiskey with him at the fire, but I didn't.

I was afraid to linger for fear I would not hear him play. I feared he would sit there for a very long time in silence. And I was too young to endure that loneliness with him. So I drove away and forgot about him.

Such is the lethal forgetting of young men.

Now, almost fifty years later, I see clearly why I drove away. I couldn't bear the thought of us both in that kitchen admitting defeat. I could not cope with what annihilation he felt when his friend did not turn up. For him it must have been a little death. A small step on the path towards silence.

There was something lovely about him and his sweet fiddle. Just like the enigmatic silence my father held when he gazed out the window in his last years or made a joke in the hospital bed or cocked his ear to the sound of a blackbird in the hospital garden as he lay between the cot sides; a kind of melancholy that awakens with age. Small moments that prefigure death and which young men will run a mile from.

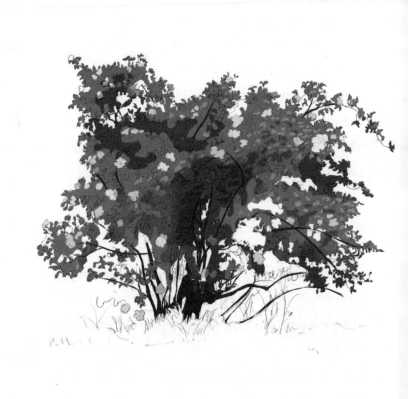

In the Lightness of Being

Getting on a plane, or taxi, and finding the first hotel in Spain, and even walking those first few days, wasn't a big deal. It didn't feel like a major decision in my life. After all, it was only for ten days. It was an incidental holiday. A bit of walking. A bit of religion-nostalgia, walking into wayside churches and looking aghast at the gaudy icons and eating lunch in the open air at wayside restaurants, and eating Spanish food in the evenings with a few glasses of wine. Who could complain about that?

But I had other expectations. I had other ideas about what great resolution or closure I might find, especially since I was subject to a regime of one heart tablet, an eye tablet, two blood pressure tablets and a couple of vitamin pills every morning. Sometimes the idea of closure, or what it might mean to resolve a life, kept me awake after dark as I lay beneath a single sheet in the warm Spanish nights and stared at the ceiling.

For me it wasn't just about dining with lovely men and women from Canada, Australia or even Japan. It wasn't just about meals with glasses of red wine.

There was walking to be done. It might even be a physical challenge at seventy, after two spinal operations.

I expected a difficult journey, and I didn't know what the end of it might reveal. Walking with my father might not be easy. And what if just thinking about him drew me back to the broken child I was long ago?

But I loved the early-morning breakfasts of cold meat and little almond cakes and hot coffee. And even though I was in love with a shadow, and obsessively haunted by the light of long-ago in Glangevlin, it didn't feel wrong.

The walk from Sarria to Santiago should have taken five days. But due to my age and medical history the travel agency was kind enough to tailor the walk to suit me. I would have ten days to complete the journey, taking no more than an average of fifteen kilometres per day, except on the last section, a journey of twenty-six kilometres which I was dreading. At least by that stage my fitness levels would have improved. Or at least that's how I assured myself in the shower each morning as I faced the dreaded carcass in the mirror.

I walked from village to village, and up the mountain and down the valleys beneath blue skies, and I kept looking forward to the moment when it would be all over: when I would finally reach the city of St James and check in for two nights at the Convento de San Francisco, a swanky hotel that used to be a convent.

I had a little camera with me on the walk. An Osmo gimble no bigger than a large cigar which captured images and video in 4K. I suppose I was fantasising about the footage on YouTube or Facebook garnishing thousands of likes. But when I examined the results after the first day's walking I was horrified at how boring it looked. Nothing more than my moving steps, my brown-clad legs and the big black Hoka shoes. And an endless number of Spanish ditches.

I had the deluded notion that thousands of people would be fascinated. But the further the Camino went on, the more I realised that the walk was extremely mundane, and there was nothing more could be said about it. Walking it is visually boring because the landscape changes slowly: hours of pathways, ditches, trees and restaurants, all visual clichés. The back of a pilgrim's head. Their legs and arms and bare shoulders. Rucksacks with water bottles bouncing on the side.

And every day was the same. Such predictability and sameness, one kilometre after the next, would be excruciating to endure online even if I was naïve enough to post such footage. And besides, the internet, YouTube, Facebook and every other form of social media was clogged, stuffed, jammed, piled with similar footage. It's as if the only people who go on the Camino are bores who like playing with their own face on screen while a few dull ditches pass behind them. I grew infuriated with Camino movies, and more infuriated with my own collection of visual clichés, and finally abandoned the camera entirely.

It was only when I stopped using it that I realised the camera had been a distraction. And earbuds and headphones were further distractions. The smartphone was a distraction.

Because to walk the Camino you need only the rhythm of the body; nothing more. You may go from one end of Galicia to the other with a phone or camera but you haven't walked the Camino. Because the real pathway is in the heart, a silent journey towards an unknown destination, and you don't get there if you don't pay attention.

Each evening I reflected on the day with a glass of wine and some food, trying to absorb the same lesson. That there is something mundane about the Camino that must be embraced. An ordinariness built into the pattern of walking that is hypnotic and to which the pilgrim must commit. And that commitment is both the process and the result.

Apart from it being good for your physical health, there is nothing more to expect. There is nothing going to happen from one day to the next. That is the insight; the marvellous revelation of walking in the lightness of being. Mentor deities are just a lens. Ultimately there is only walking and paying attention. The mentor deity dissolves into the simple reality of being. And then you're home.

Even ideas can't be sustained on a long walk. They too dissolve in the air you breathe. The body awakens and takes over. The body sweats, shits, washes, sleeps, wakes, eats, walks.

It's like swimming in a new way. It's like being a fish who discovers air. And knowing that in the ordinary we find heaven. In the mundane we find bliss. What redeemed the men of Glangevlin from their unlettered lives was that they were always walking. Even when they were still and unmoved beside the flickering flames in the stove, their hearts were walking, breathing and awake to that moment.

Walking, I realised, is a sort of chanting in the body. I was enduring a ten-day embodiment of song. The walking body was the mantra and it enveloped my awareness.

My mantra began like this: I am walking with my father. Nothing more. No expectation. No effort made to pray. No hope of surprises. My mantra had no meaning. I just walked. Remembered. Reflected. Paid attention to whatever random ghosts stumbled into my mindstream. And eventually at the end of most days, the patterns of thought, ideation, structures of meaning and disturbing emotions had all dissolved around the mantra, and the mantra had dissolved into the body, and only the body floated on the surface of being.

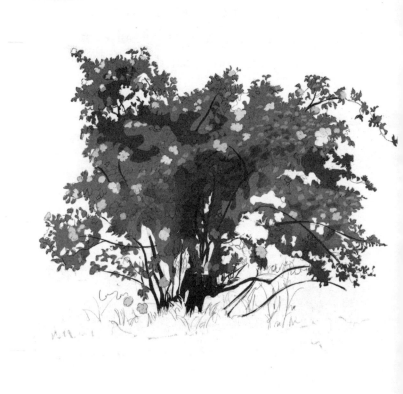

Stars Unfolding

In Glangevlin we believed in many ghosts, who stumbled around in myth and story. We spoke of wells and other magical spaces when we leaned on the counter of the Glan Bar. And we spoke with hyperbolic language and reached for poetic words to name our loneliness although we could never name it exactly. Psychobabble was a coinage not yet minted and we lived in a ghostly fog of storytelling. There were bog holes where people had been drowned. And strangers who had called to houses and taken people away that were never seen again. There were mysterious babies found under bushes or beside some well or on the steps of a church. The night was haunted by our anxieties though nobody was schooled in the psychological language that might have helped us name or understand the world. All we could do was believe in everything and hope for the best. We wondered and were bewildered by everything around us. But we understood nothing. And the drink at the bar was a comforting libation.

We lived with wind and rain and hungry sheep, with wet coats and bicycles and pot-bellied stoves. Our little pub was an architecture that provided shelter from both worldly and interior weather.

We spoke of the dead and ghosts, of Vietnam and the farts that governed us from Dublin. We watched Kojak the detective with the lollipop on the television and bemoaned the price of silage, and endlessly we brooded on the townland names, the geography of the parish, and where the names came from, and what they meant, and who lived where, and how everyone was related to everyone else, and what their nicknames were.

We spoke of the Sean Terry Joes, and the Tommy Young Andies, the Joe Mickey Ernies and the Feley Joe Feleys, and how each tribe was related. It was like reading the palm of a hand we loved. And the hand was the land itself and the cobweb of lines across the palm were the links from one family to another through marriage, birth and blood.

But love was never spoken of. For some it was on a higher plane, like divine grace, and for others it was just frightening. But one way or another love could never be contained in language. It was not allowed on the agenda of our little parliament at the bar.

The solution was music. Jigs and reels and sad love songs constituted the only commentary on love. And the subject was delegated to the musicians like they were a sub-committee with special competence in the matter. We had Frankie Arthur's fiddle, and Francie Charlie Jack's box accordion, and the sweet tenor voice of Eddie Hughie Hughdie.

There was no avoiding the full moon or the snow-capped mountain peak or the far-flung glory of the Milky Way. There was no denying the mysterious shadows around the Shannon Pot, the bubbling well in the night. It would have been superfluous to reduce those grandeurs to debate. It would have been impossible to live in the landscape without awe and tenderness. But only music could express the depth of our love for the world around us.

How could I forget the night of the party in Joe Pheadar's house to welcome his sister the nun home from America for a few weeks. And how could I not celebrate with everyone else, even if I had buried my father the same day.

A nun with a beautiful face, high saintly cheekbones and wide blue eyes, as slim as a dancer; her expression implied something heroic and chaste, and full of integrity like an eagle.

Beneath a black veil she smiled and spoke to me with deliciously soft syllables. Her sharp American vowels churned in the rich buttery accent of her homeland and blended into sentences that fell on me like an elegant blanket of music. Speaking loudly, her voice carried the colour of years spent in the Bronx, but when she spoke quietly to me I could hear in the whispering all the warm syllables of Glangevlin.

I was only twenty-two. Young enough to be amazed by her vast experience, her long fingers and the fact that she too was an older woman who gazed at me like she might have been my sister in a former life. She could see to the heart of me.

All the elder women of Glangevlin were like sisters or mothers to me. They knew the ropes. How to make love, give birth, put up with men and remain in good humour. And they liked men. They lit up when men came into the room. They teased and taunted men, and sometimes could release a flash of anger that would send a shiver up any male spine. They knew the secret pathways to joy and could reveal where treasures lay hidden.

But the nun was different. Adorned with a veil, focused as an eagle, there was some kind of generosity in the way she spoke and smiled. And she was quick-witted and could exchange bawdy jibes with the other women without any problem. But it was her gaze that drew my attention. Even years afterwards, when I discovered the writings of Julian of Norwich, I immediately thought of that nun.

Julian of Norwich was locked in a room as an anchorite until her death, had a cat for the mice and a window to the world outside for listening to pilgrims' problems, and in times of plague and war had one basic message – that all will be well. She stared at the dead cadaver of Christ on the cross in her visions, and if the hagiographers are to be believed, she endured many visions and ecstasies.

So, she must have had an exceptional mental strength, and when I read her, and thought about her, I would see the face of that nun from long ago. Serenity was embedded in her expression like it might have been etched in stone.

It was just one of those faces I could never forget.

'My father was buried today,' I told her. She took my hand and squeezed it in the usual gesture of sympathy, but it felt different than any other handshake. She looked at me while she held it. Her eyes enormous brown pools of attention.

'I was studying for the priesthood,' I declared, for no particular reason, 'but I only lasted a year.'

She nodded her head, as if she understood all the failures in life a young man might have to endure. From my brief encounter with her in that moment I felt the night was different from all other nights. She was different from all other women. And my father had just died.

In the lounge of the Glan Bar, where I first

laid eyes on her before the party, the nun was surrounded by other women. Annie Joe served in the mineral bar in the hall and was always full of advice about who I should dance with. Rosie and Maya were sisters from Donegal. They married Glangevlin men in Scotland and then ended up in the mountains of west Cavan. They too helped in the bar, which is why I'd met them earlier that night in the storeroom where they were drinking mugs of tea. It was customary at a dance to make tea and sandwiches for the band so that the musicians could have supper afterwards.

The two women were in the storeroom behind the mineral bar. The place was stacked with crates of lemonade and fizzy orange bottles. They turned on a geyser for tea and made the sandwiches and then passed the rest of the evening until the end of the dance chatting. I was exhausted from the ordeal of my father's funeral when I arrived in the door.

I crawled up on the crates and drew my overcoat across my chest and went to sleep. It was a cradling my little soul required. My father not cold in his grave, and me stretched on the crates, falling into magical slumber.

But after a few minutes they woke me, reminding me that I was in the storeroom, and saying I couldn't sleep there and that I should go to the pub.

'It's only nine o'clock,' they said. 'It's too early to be falling asleep. Why don't you go down to the pub and have a drink.'

So, I went down to the Glan Bar, about five minutes away in a car. The area to the fore of the pub, and the back yard, and even the area in front of the post office was packed with tractors, vans, jeeps and a few other terminally ill saloon cars. There were lights on in the lounge. And the bar was so full that I found it difficult to prise open the door even just to get inside. Someone was leaning up against it on the inside and wouldn't budge.

I hoped that the fun would banish the numbness I had been feeling since the undertaker had closed the lid on my father's coffin.

And fortunately, there was music in the lounge that night. Frankie Arthur played 'The Battering

Ram' and 'The Swallow's Tail'. Eddie Hughie Hughdie sang 'Spancil Hill' and 'The Shores of Lough Erne'. Rose, the landlady, and Vesty, her brother, dodged in and out between the young farmers who were sitting in overcoats on small stools. Every low table was stacked with pints of beer and glasses of Babycham and from a dozen ashtrays the smoke of old butts rose to the ceiling. Perfume wafted off girls in the furthest corners away from the fire, as they huddled together in party dresses and tried to keep reasonably cool. Along the side wall the nun and her family proudly shook hands with every new customer that darkened the door.

'Are you coming back to the house later?' the nun asked.

It was summer. There was little darkness. Everyone was on holidays drinking and singing and making music in the lounge for as long as they could and then most would go round to Joe Pheadar's house for what was euphemistically called 'the tea'. Such was the style of parties.

The women were slim in their dresses and jeans and the men were gaunt rakes even after a feed of pints and there was always two or three standing at the door of the lounge, half in and half out, not sure if they should stay in the bar of old smoky men or edge further into the dizzy field of frocks and girls that dominated the lounge; men bewildered by the feminine glow of young factory workers who had purses full of money. They stood at the door like they did in church on Sundays, almost afraid to enter the sacred space. They stood like whippets, and everyone was ravenous for food and showed no restraint when Vesty and Rose arrived with long trays of ham and chicken sandwiches and large mugs of tea.

If the long months of winter darkness were an extended sigh of despair in the darkness, then those eight weeks of summer were always an antidote; an endless flow of music, drink and exuberant *sean-nós* dancing. And no one paid the slightest attention to the clock.

So everyone was going to the party. Even me, since I had already been invited.

The Glangevlin way of making tea was to place loose leaves in a teapot that had been sitting on the range for ten minutes and had been scalded with boiling water. In the absence of a teapot or when making tea for a large number of people a spoon of loose tea was placed in each mug before the infusion with boiling water from the kettle or, if it were in the hall, a geyser.

I imagined the loose tea might cause the brew to thicken like tar in the cup but the leaves always fell to the bottom, the milk was always measured perfectly and water from the well always drew out the most exquisite taste that tea could produce.

I was still pondering the party and should I go or not. Considering that my father had just been buried, it might have been appropriate to say I was in mourning and head home alone. On the other hand, there would be music and recitations and whiskey in Joe Pheadar's and there was one girl I longed for and I had spent weeks figuring out how I might get talking to her. The fact that she was a relation of the nun and certain to be at the party clinched it for me.

That's when I spoke to the nun, mentioning my father, and adding my little story about having been in a seminary for a year when I was eighteen.

I suppose I thought that would make a connection between us.

And thus, she asked me to the house. It was brief and simple and I went off to order a pint in the bar, and the music played in the lounge, and eventually the nun and her entourage left, and the crowd thinned out as it did every night, and when closing time came I ventured round the roads through rushes and bushes and winding laneways to the door of Joe Pheadar's two-storey farmhouse. From the open front door there was no doubt that neighbours had been in the kitchen all evening erecting sandwiches like skyscrapers on blue-patterned dinner plates and ensuring that there were large black kettles boiling on the range. And the sweet smell of bog turf permeated the house.

The nun squeezed my hand once again, welcoming me to the house she was reared in, and thanked me for coming as if it were a compliment to her that I should turn up. And when the tea and sandwiches were finished someone began a conversation about the fair in Dowra and about neighbours who had been recently laid to rest in the graveyard. And when words failed and the silence stretched long enough for an intoxicated guest to raise the first notes of a song, it could have been said that the party was warming up and the night was but a pup.

One song and one recitation and maybe three or four tunes on the box, and then the pattern repeated again. Until a fiddle or flute was taken from the boot of a car outside and the collective emotion moved up a notch.

It may have been one in the morning when the woman I had been dreaming of appeared at the door, took her portion of tea and a bottle of beer, and after a modicum of chat with the nun beside the range she ended up on a stool next to me.

Then she leaned over and said, 'Will you leave me home later?'

I knew she wasn't just looking for a taxi. It was a code. Young ladies used it all the time in bars and dancehalls; it was a useful and direct way for the girl to choose her boy and force him into a small commitment without implying any partiality on her part.

But we remained on our stools and showed no sign of hurry, until I had heard enough song and drunk enough whiskey and until she had talked to her friends and relations for a long time. Then separately we both vanished into the night, so fast that nobody would have noticed we were leaving together. Down the hills and up the hills, around the bends and left at the crossroads, until she said, 'Will we go up and look at the pot?'

It was a bright night and Cuilcagh mountain was a dense black presence above which the full moon was clear and sharp against the sky. The moon swallowed the light of the stars, and only the plough was faint above Fermanagh. The huge moon so radiant in the sky on its journey east that it flooded the world with enough light to find our pathway through the fields, and the woman beside me was transformed as we stood in the bushes and battered our way to the water's edge.

'Don't go near or you might fall in,' she teased.

The Shannon Pot is rarely still. The water shimmers even on days with no wind, because the water welling from below never ceases. And yet on this night the surface was completely still. The test is always if you can see the moon unfractured in the water. This is probably caused by excessive amounts of water flowing up from below in wet weather, or seeping down through the limestone from lakes higher up the mountain, causing the surface to appear still. But for us wrapped in mythic wonder, the stillness implied that no water was flowing, and the well was sleeping.

We could see the moon. And seeing the moon in the water had an effect on us I could not explain.

What more awesome use of the human eye could there be than to gaze at a full moon, a pallid glow above the mountain, giving forth this light for us to find our way through the marsh and bog and ditch en route from the car at the edge of the road.

The moon was deep inside the pool. The pool was holding it and presenting it to us.

But I felt sad. There was something distracting me from the woman beside me. Someone who could have been the beloved of my life if only I paid attention in this moment. We were young and enjoyed singing in kitchens. But who knows what we might have become together if that moment had opened in the right manner. If we had seen in each other the same moon. But it didn't happen. And then the moment passed.

Almost immediately I blamed the nun because she was so beautiful that I had been mesmerised as I watched her at the party. I idolised her veil, the serenity in her face, the clarity of her uniform proclaiming her devotion, and maybe I thought that such was the path I too should follow. Alternatively, I might have concluded that the woman I was with was not my true beloved. Not the one I drank the wine with before the grapes were grown, as Rumi might say. But one way or another, I quit my teaching job and returned to the seminary a few months later. And my conviction is that neither woman was the cause.

I knew my father was the reason that I turned again to find a father-god. The assault on my senses at the funeral left an emptiness in me so raw that I couldn't fill it with anything else. Through his death I was tethered to my father for life, because he was buried in the same clay that waited for me. They say that you can only love when you understand. And if someone had asked me who my father was I would have just said he is dead. But that at least was a way of understanding him. He was an absence in my heart. I could say I loved him now.

In grief a person can uncover fresh emotions that will endure for decades. The casual glance of a saintly nun, or the turning away from a lover, can close the door of the heart for years. But to find understanding, and from understanding to embrace love, is a journey that can only be described as the path of wisdom.

So it was with me ever since I looked into the coffin and saw my daddy in his blue suit, his full set of teeth in place and his black-rimmed spectacles at his side. I was fortunate.

And fortunate also because the two women in the parish hall, drinking mugs of tea and guarding the sandwiches, had not banished me. They guided me to the pub. And the nun's big eyes were as clear as if she were an angel come from the pure land. And the woman I longed for had not sat down by accident. There are no accidents. The universe unfolds like a rose, a fact that is obvious to anyone who stands in the night beneath a mountain with the Milky Way stretched above.

Everything has meaning when I see it with the eye of the heart. Everything leads to some destination. I thought the moon would clinch it. The moon would fix me for life. I'd be telling this story decades later to my grandchildren, how my life had changed in an instant. But it was my father I was destined to love in that moment. Because I suddenly understood him. *He is the absence inside me now*, I thought. And I felt the weight of love for the first time in my life. All because I understood. He was gone. A kind of empty space, a cavity of darkness in the heart that left me sore and wounded. It made me normal. I was empty too. I was like him. A dead moon inside me.

And no wonder that wells and holy wells became a kind of melancholic refuge for me down the years; places where the moon is never found and where the water holds the dark and sings only of emptiness. Even fifty years later, there are nights when I get out of bed if I can't sleep and walk where the moon leads me down to a cliff from where I can see the lake and see the moon reflected in the lake. I walk through the woodland and the garden and find the same moon drenching the leaves. I stare at it and know the moon to be the same single moon I met on that night long ago. And I wish that after fifty years I might still find him in my heart. Still know Daddy as a presence, beautiful as the moon on the lake, singing its song of praise to the universe.

PART TWO

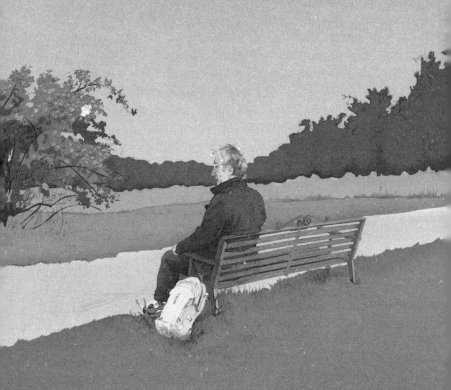

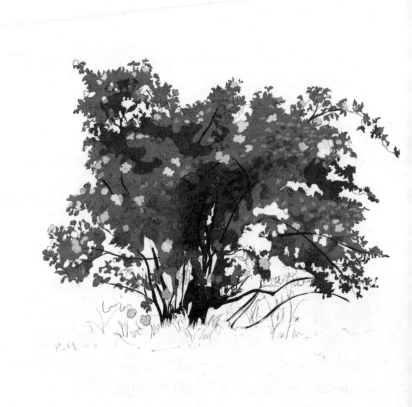

The Pilgrim Path

From Morgade to Portomarin was a lovely walk. I had overcome several problems, most notably the footwear. The Hoka shoes were a mistake. I bought them in Letterkenny the week before I left for Spain. They cost 270 euro. My jaw dropped when the salesperson declared the price, but I had researched the shoe and from everything I'd read I believed these magical soft-cushioned soles were the right option. Soles as thick as planks of wood and gauze-like uppers. Perhaps I should have spent more time breaking them in before the long walk. Or perhaps they were designed for keeping someone comfortable when standing for long hours but not necessarily for trekking.

Anyway, after the first twenty kilometres three of my toes were wounded, each from being squashed against the other, and on the knuckle of the big toe which had swelled considerably in two days there was a deep blister. A sea of pus beneath the surface.

And then that broke.

I went to a *farmacia* in Ventas de Narón when I arrived in town and put antiseptic cream on the wound, then a plaster, and finally a little cylinder of spongey foam between each toe to isolate them and prevent them rubbing together. The following morning, I could only manage to limp five kilometres down the road before I had to change the bandages and the foam cushions between the toes.

I didn't believe I would make it to Palas that day, although it was only twelve kilometres, and when I got there I went to a gift shop, bought a pair of sandals for twenty-eight euro, got rid of the bandages and socks, and felt reasonably comfortable all afternoon. The following morning, I wore the sandals again, tying the Hoka shoes to the back strap of my rucksack, and I walked in comfort for the entire day, covering fifteen kilometres to Melide.

Yellow arrows on the streets and pavements directed me through the town and out into lush countryside, with green fields and tall trees each side of a wide tarred laneway. But it might as well have been Ireland. Without the drama of sore toes, the walking was still mantric; a rhythm that ingrained itself deeper and deeper in my mind-stream. I wondered how I would ever be able to stop. Maybe just walking with no destination, with no expectations and with no narrative is the true nature of our souls.

I walked without knowing or seeing. I crossed little rivers, zig-zagged through mud, hopped across stone stiles, low stone walls, but I was not in the mundane world now. I had fallen into an imaginal realm. Evagrius, the old wise monk of the desert in the early church, might have under-stood this as walking into the darkness of God's embrace, and Marilynne Robinson might have called it paying attention to an eternal presence. But I wasn't that far on at this stage. I was still walking with sore toes, and sometimes worried if I might need to use a toilet suddenly when I was walking through suburbia.

I noticed sounds more than thoughts. I could hear bees sometimes, and the wind moving through reeds and the branches of trees above me. I could hear solitary cars in the distance and the frenzy of a thousand cars each time I came into a town. I could hear voices of other humans rising out of restaurants and cafés and in market squares. I could hear water in the distance, and then closer as I approached a lively stream or waterfall. I could hear the sound of other pilgrims, their feet pushing on over gravel pathways, their breath pushing in and out as they passed beside me.

I remember one afternoon in Arzúa, a town en route and halfway to Santiago, I lay stretched on the bed with sore limbs considering all these things. I had been walking for three hours and it was now 2 p.m. The weather clock outside the *farmacia* said 29°C. Each day was hotter, but the morning had been pleasant under a canopy of huge trees and the scent of eucalyptus in the air for miles.

I was close enough now to Santiago to feel confident I would make it, and the feet had healed wonderfully in the cheap sandals. I was even tempted to leave the Hokas in a church porch or give them to a charity shop if I passed one. But considering the price I paid for them, and with my Cavan common sense, I kept them tied to the rucksack; in the right context I might still get some benefit from them back in Ireland.

So, I showered and lay on the bed in my hotel, listening to noises from a courtyard down below where people were having lunch.

When I looked out the window, I saw a man of about my own age, in a white suit and straw hat. He was sitting at a table below me and facing away from me, so all I could see was his back, the suit and the straw hat on the top of his head. I could see the old brown hands like thick ivy swatting flies and tapping the table as he waited and raising the little glass of wine to his lips.

But otherwise he was very still and when he spoke his voice sounded sharp and humourless. He was talking to a woman, who might have been his daughter. And she was minding two young boys who were playing in the flower beds that skirted the stone walls of the yard.

The man seemed to be chastising her, his hands flying in the air, his fists punching the table, his head bobbing this way and that beneath his white straw hat. And she was taking it with a smile, as if it was all okay. She nibbled at her spaghetti with a fork, in between glances at the two boys, curbing their desires to tear the roses down with their boots and climb the wall.

But it was the suit that the old man wore in the courtyard that absorbed me. It hung on him as on a skeleton and I could only think of my father in the coffin, when his corpse was clad in Tom McKenna's finest tailoring.

I had been so used to my father naked beneath the sheets of various hospital beds that I had forgotten what he looked like when he was fully dressed. And then in the morgue, when I gazed into the coffin, he appeared more alive than his usual self in a remarkable blue suit.

One day a few years before he retired, my father ordered a new suit from Tom McKenna, the main outfitter for gentlemen in Cavan town, and when he returned from the measuring ceremony that evening he announced to his wife that the suit would be blue.

'Blue?' she exclaimed, slightly horrified. She had married a man who wore grey suits. What would he be doing in a blue one? What for that matter would any man be doing in a blue suit in 1964?

'Actually,' he said, 'Mr McKenna says it will look much the same as a grey suit. It *is* a grey suit. But they call it blue.'

'Did you see the material?' she wondered.

'No,' he admitted, 'I'm not good on colours.'

The reason I recall that blue suit is because it completed him in the coffin. He looked well.

In the early sixties there was an air of change everywhere. Young people wore long hair and people gossiped about the possibility of colour televisions coming to Ireland, like they had in America.

So, Mr McKenna convinced my father that the dark charcoal grey was a thing of the past. 'Men are wearing brighter colours nowadays,' he explained, and to his surprise, my father agreed.

'Give me the blue,' my father said, and so it was made up in a few weeks. There was no waistcoat with it. Apparently, Mr McKenna said that waistcoats too were a thing of the past. Everything will be casual in the years ahead. And there was a place for a belt on the trousers, although that's where my father drew the line. He believed in braces; it was a moral stand against the impending decline of civilisation and what he saw as the onslaught of dances originating in the rhythms of Africa.

Belts might be acceptable to young gyrating teenagers who desired nothing but hedonistic orgies in dens of iniquity described as 'night clubs', but not to him.

On Christmas Day of that year, he wore the suit with braces to the dining table. We had no guests to liven things up. There was nothing unusual about the food. It was the standard feast of Yuletide joy cooked with stress and tension by my mother in the kitchen.

And when we sat down to eat, my father took off the jacket and tossed it on the chair. My mother chastised him for not hanging it up with the coats under the stairs. They argued about why it was not appropriate to hang a suit among the over-coats, and then fell silent for the afternoon.

From that day until he went into hospital to die, I never saw him wear anything else in public other than the blue suit.

But even in those cameo scenes, composites in my memory, fictions assembled from multiple

Christmas meals, I find it difficult to remember him at will, until I see some old man that triggers my memory, like the man in the white suit below my hotel window.

My father was a diminutive figure and had not the capacity to bully. He was never abusive or drunk, and I saw him cry in the kitchen one day as he described the endless bullying he experienced in the county council office where he worked. There was one colleague who knew of his humble beginnings and used the details as a licence to undermine and sneer at him. It's possible that these were the kind of things that isolated him, his fear of being shamed driving his remoteness and his reticence to be even slightly flamboyant in his dress.

I would venture into his solitude sometimes, when he was sitting with his newspaper under the lamp in the drawing room, and try to make conversation. I would talk about ideas that I knew fascinated him; the idea of God was never far away.

He showed no interest in politics or sport. And there is no evidence that he liked dogs, cats or other animals.

My father was always in danger of losing his balance due to his thick glasses lenses and therefore the idea of the cat dodging in and out under his feet was a non-starter. So the cat never got beyond the kitchen door when father was about, and I suspected that my mother's coldness towards the cat was also some kind of loyalty to her husband rather than coming from her own heart, as I had seen a picture of her as a teenager standing with her brother Oliver in the back yard of the pub in Castlepollard clutching a big black cat so tightly that one might suppose she loved it fiercely.

It's not that my father ever declared himself against cats. But I think my mother internalised his authority and noted his displeasure even without him venting it. She became an extension of him, sometimes rising to contempt for the cat as if on his behalf.

I didn't need Spanish to know the man in the courtyard below my window. I had him sussed. Here was the iron authority of a patriarch, the man whose word is final. The one who has been to the university of life, and ultimately holds all intellectuals in contempt because he knows that ideology doesn't butter parsnips or put olive oil on the bread. He knows it's all about survival and the joy is in the wine with family and children. The rest of the world doesn't matter. Philosophy or ideas are but dangerous flirtations with the devil.

I was projecting a lot of stuff onto the back of another man's head, whose face I couldn't even see. But he was not my father. He was just a man in a suit. It wasn't even an impeccably tailored suit, but you could tell by the way he wore it on his shoulders that he thought it was. And after many hours and many kilometres walking with my father, I was beginning to remember more of the past. I began to see him more clearly in my mind. And as the man's white suit in the courtyard drew me back to my father in a blue suit, so the blue suit drew me further back to other suits he wore when I was younger.

My father wore dark suits. A charcoal grey sometimes with a faint pinstripe which had a run-down feel to it. He presented as a clerk of lesser importance, though he was never without his Parker pen, a plump little submarine with a burgundy belly sitting in his breast pocket. The silver upper half with its Parker logo beamed from that position on his breast pocket where a man might pin war medals.

The Parker pen was perhaps a nod to something private and personal; the poverty of his youth, perhaps, when the nib of a school pen got lodged in his hip during an altercation with another boy and his grandmother was called to attend him and bring him to the Royal Hospital in Donnybrook where nurses extracted the nib.

Or perhaps the Parker pen was a trophy he cherished in remembrance of all the years he spent by candlelight and gaslight in a Dublin boarding house trying to understand the meaning of numbers in his accountancy correspondence courses. Whatever the reason, the Parker pen became his talisman, the working tool of an accountant and a comforting symbol of meaning as he struggled through books of Catholic apologetics.

Apart from the Parker pen he was just a man in a dull suit, and far from drawing attention to himself, people in his company were inclined to presume he was some kind of servant or doorman. The other professional classes who lived beside us mocked him for his airs and graces. For this was a man who had nowhere to hide from the sneers of well-heeled university graduates in the deeply divided class society of Ireland in the 1950s, unless he guarded his story and kept to himself.

As my imagination tossed up these possibilities I began to see his face again, as it was sometime long ago when I was young, and for the first time it seemed more frightened than formidable. Was it that he had just so much shame to cover up, so much devastation in his family? The drinking father, the deceased mother, the old grandmother trying to rule the two-roomed cottage with an iron fist. His dancing uncle who did turns in all the music halls.

And then with what ruthlessness did he leave his grandmother, when his sister died of TB in her teens, his father deceased and his uncle married? The granny was alone and he was in Clare, desperate to create for himself a life far away from all that poverty.

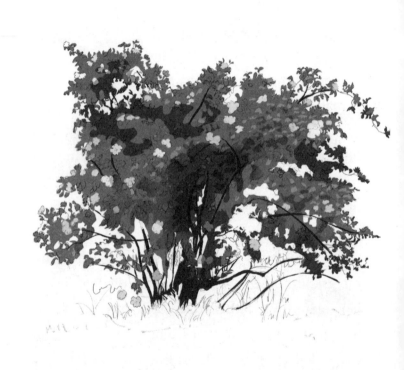

Suits and Scholars

I grew up in the 1960s, and to me the suit and tie and burgundy Parker pen were the accoutrements of lost empires. Like the young people around me at that time, I was living on the edge of a radical new dawn. Our lives appeared so important to us compared to those who had gone before us. Our casual clothes, long hair, sandals and patchouli oil, even as we hitched the highways and byways of Ireland in the late sixties, on our way to various folk festivals up and down the country, were the uniform of a burgeoning cultural revolution.

I wore the uniform. I had long hair, denim jeans and large colourful shirts. In summer I wore sandals, shorts and colourful vests. Even as an ordained priest in the 1980s I proclaimed my faith in liberation theology, a preferential option for the poor masking raw Marxist ideology and vehemently opposed to the capitalist church of the past and all its trappings such as antiquated liturgies. As a curate and school-teacher I dressed in salmon-coloured trousers and a white blouse-like shirt with ruffles at the shoulders when I went to teach religion to young boys and girls in a Fermanagh grammar school or as I swaggered around the houses of the elderly bringing them the body of Christ in communion and lots of gossip. Even from the very beginning of my short ministry in the church I was on a search for spaces of dissent. When I was appointed chaplain to a nursing home run by nuns in Cork for three months in the summer of 1981 I dressed in more lavish and brightly coloured shirts and jeans, cycling round the city with the wind in my face.

I drank in Counihan's in the centre of town and in The Long Valley, lunching on doorstep sand-wiches of bacon or roast beef. I cycled from the nursing home in Montenotte on summer evenings down the hills to MacCurtain Street and across the bridge into Patrick Street, wearing the same high-quality white shirt and pink trousers as was my uniform everywhere. It was a delight to resist the black priestly garments of my profession and wander through the bohemian wonderland of students and artists. I was at the cutting edge of resistance.

And the more often I could use the word 'resistance' the better, when I was chatting up women in The Long Valley. My life was resistance. My vision of the church was resistance. My bicycle was resistance. Capitalist shite just had to be resisted.

And working in a nursing home for the elderly I encountered capitalist shite daily. So, I felt validated as a priest not by virtue of the church's claim that Jesus might set you free and give you peace, but rather by virtue of my 'resistance'.

It was all very easy in Cork, among so many students in so many bars. And The Long Valley was the best of them for meeting students.

But Counihan's was an entirely different kettle of fish. It was situated beyond the post office, towards the South Mall, and was another world entirely. The floorboards creaked. The furniture had been gathered from the pages of some bleak novel about Ireland in the 1950s.

A shaded counter, with slivers of light coming in from a small window where Mr Counihan sat on a high stool behind the bar, gazing out at the street and philosophising on the human condition. A shaft of light crossed his chest but left his face in shadow. His wife appeared occasionally with mugs of tea and sandwiches. And on the customer side of the bar, there were hardly more than three or four men murmuring into pints of stout in the early evenings when I was wont to visit.

So, it was a stunning surprise when I found the place jammed with academics, and students with satchels, one evening; long hair, sideburns, cigarettes, pints wrestled from the bar and everyone in a state of agitation. The distinguished academic David Norris sweating in an open-neck shirt. Anthony Burgess, the illustrious English writer, scowling at a young woman and blowing the smoke of a long, thin cigar into her face.

It was James Joyce's birthday centenary and there had been a symposium somewhere earlier on the university campus and the academic and the writer had been in attendance. Now here was I, absorbing the banter and arguments and the erudition of these great scholars still in debate about detailed passages of the great text.

The following Saturday afternoon I happened to return to the same shaded place, ordered a pint and positioned myself at the counter, angled towards the window, while three men drank on the long side of the counter. Mr Counihan was silent as he pulled my pint of Guinness. He stared out the window, allowing the half-full pint glass to settle before finishing it off. He muttered to himself.

'Absent friends,' he said. 'Absent friends. Isn't that the truth?'

I didn't know what he meant.

'They were all toasting absent friends on Thursday night,' he explained.

'Oh right,' I said. 'Yes.' Remembering that they had on a few occasions toasted Joyce with the phrase.

'Great writers indeed,' said Mr Counihan.

'Yes,' I agreed, wondering why he was focusing on me.

'You're an educated man,' he said as he put the pint in front of me. 'So tell me this: how many great writers are there in this country?'

The customers leaned into the bar and sneered.

'A great question,' one of them declared.

I confessed my ignorance.

'Ah, you must know,' Mr Counihan insisted. 'I mean, if you were to take the whole of Ireland over the past century, how many great writers would you say we could claim?'

I had no idea.

'Well,' he said, 'there was Joyce. And Yeats. Maybe Synge?'

I didn't budge.

'I'd say there was about a dozen of them in all,' he concluded. And the chorus of men listening agreed. Yes, they all thought about a dozen.

'Yes,' I said, 'I suppose that's about right. A dozen. That would be about right, Mr Counihan.'

'Yes,' he said, 'it's about right.' Taking my shillings from the counter for the drink, dropping the pennies into the till one by one and closing the till with a tingling bang for effect.

'About a dozen,' he declared, his voice now rising to the cadences of a barrister in the district court. 'And do you know this,' he finished, 'half of them drink in here on Saturdays.'

As far as I can remember, Anthony Burgess was dressed in a white linen suit on the night in question. David Norris wore a pinstripe though he had discarded the jacket.

When I returned to the bar and Mr Counihan shared his astute observation regarding local poets in Cork, it struck me that he wasn't saying anything derogatory about the distinguished guests who had come in their suits from Dublin and London. It was the local icons of bohemia that failed to impress him. And me too, since I was dressed like a Corkonian Goth. I wanted to be a poet with faded jeans and my hair in a mess. But in Counihan's I had met two very distinguished writers, and both wore suits.

All the way home I thought of my father in his suit, and how conservative he was and how he too had tried to be a writer. He took meticulous care with every book review he wrote. David Marcus in *The Irish Press* would send him history books and books with some religious connection. A biography about the Nun of Kenmare fascinated him. And books about de Valera. But it was when Malcolm Muggeridge, the distinguished English Catholic intellectual, wrote him a brief personal letter thanking him for a review of Muggeridge's book *Jesus Rediscovered* that I saw his hand tremble and his eyes almost frightened with tears as if he had in some way truly made it as a writer. Or at least from beginnings in poverty and illiteracy and no formal education, that was as good as it was going to get.

I pushed my bike up the hill that Saturday evening to Montenotte and chained it to the drainpipe outside the chaplain's house where I was working; delighted and exhausted by the assumption that I was in any way part of the literary cohort that was flocking around the great Joycean scholars. I lay on the lawn staring up at the moon and feeling more joy than I had felt since my father died five years earlier. Then I went inside and upstairs to the bedroom and rummaged in the wardrobe for my own suit. I put it on, not because I suddenly wanted to look like a conservative cleric but because I wanted to be my father. I wanted to identify with his style; to belong in the grammar of his clothes. To write as he had written. And to succeed where he had failed, because his failure was to have been born poor.

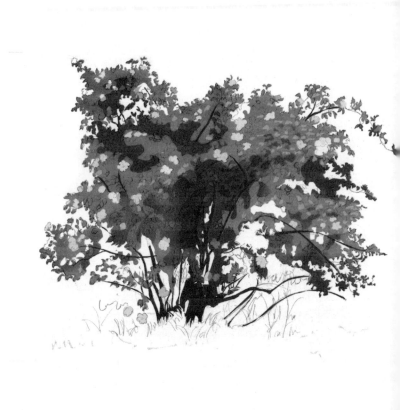

The Pilgrim's Muesli

Approaching the town of Salceda in the mid-afternoon sun, for the last stop before the bit that was terrifying me, the twenty-six-kilometre trek to Santiago, I was wiped out. My feet were the only thing not stinging with pain. My back felt like there were nettles inside my spine. My hips were numb, and my arse and guts felt as if they were made of stone. But I wasn't unduly alarmed. The surgeon in Beaumont three years earlier had said that the nerves are the slowest thing of all to heal. And he was right, although I recall him advising me to be cautious and patient with the healing process and not overdo the exercise. I was still on one gabapentin tablet per day to keep the nerves calm and I just upped the dose on days when the nerves in my back and legs were demanding too much attention. On the road to

Salceda by late afternoon I had taken my third tablet.

But the real problem was the *albergue* booked for me. Firstly, it was outside the town. This meant an extra two kilometres' walking. And when I got there, they had no knowledge of the booking. In fact, I was at the wrong hotel, and there was no way I could walk back into town.

'Do you have anything at all?' I pleaded with the receptionist, a slim lady with dark brown eyes behind round spectacles.

She looked unhappy and a bit constipated for a moment as she flicked through the book on the desk.

'No. We have no vacancies.'

'Can you call me a taxi?' I asked.

But by the time it arrived and took me to the original hotel I was exhausted. These were the small distractions I had not prepared for when measuring how I might manage the Camino. And when I finally showered and lay on a bed in my hotel that evening, I was so dehydrated and tired that I skipped food and fell into a deep sleep.

I woke hours later, around midnight, to the warm sensation of urine around my groin. I leaped up, pulled the sheets back, ran to the bathroom, a horror dawning on me that I had wet the bed.

This was a catastrophe, but it was not long after midnight, so I had time to sort it out. The cause of the accident was my post-operative condition: severe numbness that had settled on my gut and groin from dehydration and exhaustion. The sheets were wet but the mattress was dry. The sheets could be left stretched over chairs with the window open while I slept in pyjamas underneath a single blanket.

It worked well. Forty minutes later I settled down to sleep. At dawn I piled the sheets into the bathroom so that the staff would know they were soiled. And I went for breakfast.

Which is where I met the Irish man. I had noticed him the previous evening standing at reception when I was checking in. An elderly man with a mop of long grey hair tied at the neck in a ponytail. A small Irish flag was sewn into the back of his rucksack, and another little tricolour adorned the flap of his breast pocket. He greeted me in a Dublin accent. As if we were old friends.

'Hello.'

'How are you?'

'Are you from Ireland?'

'Yes.'

'We must talk later.'

'Yes. Definitely.'

But then I forgot about him, until breakfast.

He waved from his seat by the window and I waved back as I collected a bowl of muesli, fruit, a plate of scrambled egg and a Spanish rasher from the buffet. I would have joined him but I was too traumatised from the accident in my room, so I got a table to myself at the window and tried to eat without too much stress. I turned on my phone screen and began reading as if I was desperately concerned about something in the news.

Having an accident at night is not something that is easy to share. I could happily dine out on all my illnesses and hospital dramas, but any hint of incontinence feels shameful; it's too personal. It's too much information. It's not like a broken leg or a heart attack. Those are heroic, manly flaws.

But pissing in the bed is a catastrophe I'd prefer to walk away from and forget.

On the way out of town there was a wayside church of cold stone, flickering candles and garish saints where people were gathering and gawking around inside and then emerging to open their rucksacks at the low stone wall surrounding the church, and drinking bottled water or in some cases having their first snack of chocolate or apple for the day.

People inside took off their sunglasses to gaze at the statues but most just gawked. They weren't devotional Christians, apart from a blind man in a wheelchair who was manoeuvred around by a woman I presumed to be his daughter. A white walking cane rested on his knees, and he wore heavy black sunglasses. And he maintained his head high as if he were visually scrutinising the world. She whispered something in his ear and then left him positioned towards the altar while she went to a statue of the Virgin Mary and lit two candles.

Her faith as it manifested in her devout gesture of blessing herself and lighting the candle, and the affection with which she attended the elderly man, moved me to imitate her.

I too stepped forward towards the statue, dropped two euro into the mouth of the collection box and lit my two candles, thinking of both my father and mother as I completed the gesture. I blessed myself as attentively as I could and I noticed the Irish man again, sitting with considerable serenity in one of the pews, his back as straight as a rod and his head up as if he was enjoying the radiance of the saint flowing down at him. His eyes were closed. He might as well have been in ecstasy. And despite his age he was clearly experiencing the walk as an enriching meditation. All I could do as I fretted over my own little issues was to envy him his tranquillity. And his physical agility.

I went out into the sunlight, placing my little yellow rucksack on the low stone wall in order to get my bottle of drinking water.

Even sucking the bottle of water at these resting points along the way felt like an act of communion.

When I was rummaging for water in my rucksack two lockets on a chain fell out. One was a golden locket in the shape of a giant almond that opened and closed. A love locket which in earlier centuries would have contained images of the betrothed pair. I don't know if the locket ever contained an image of my mother or father, but I knew it was from him to her because the words spoke the truth.

'To Nellie with Love.'

The phrase was inscribed on the back with the date: a certain month in 1950. I found it after she died in 2012. I had kept it on my desk, as scholars once kept skulls beside their books to remind them of the shortness of life.

In the eloquent calligraphy of her name, I imagined his excitement on that date. On that very date in time. It wasn't for her birthday or Christmas or for any other public occasion that I could discern. It was an arbitrary day in August of 1950 that must have meant something particular to both. It implied some intimacy. Not a necessary ritual or duty, but an extra gesture, a flourish of poetry to say something to her. And she treasured it clearly to her end.

But I had thrown it in the bottom of the rucksack when I was packing, as a talisman, a symbol of remembrance, and I felt it was auspicious that it fell out just after I had emerged from the church. The coincidence allowed me to construe significance and meaning into the locket; and I suppose that too is how religion works.

There is a phrase that monastics in Russian monasteries were fond of: they would say that 'when the student is ready, the teacher will appear'.

It's as if religion sustains in us an openness to the poetry of accidental patterns, and the meaning we need can sometimes be embodied in the casual bric-a-brac of a mundane world.

The locket surfaced after I had lit two candles. There was nothing magical in that, apart from the poetic shape that I imposed on the details. But I now felt blessed. And I was confident that it would not be long now before the teacher appeared. Because after the humiliation of the night and the quiet balm of the little church with its cool flagstones and flickering light in the shadows, I was ready for walking.

Just then the blind man passed me, his daughter pushing the wheelchair, the sunglasses covering his eyes, the white cane across his knees, and beads of sweat on her brow as she pushed him towards a waiting taxi. And I held the locket from 1950 in the palm of my hand and walked on.

The wet sheets and the shame of my incontinence also brought a stark memory of my father to mind. I don't ever remember him being incontinent in the bed but he kept the chamber pot close.

He retired in 1968 and every morning he breakfasted from a tray that my mother carried to the bedroom. He insisted on squeezed oranges. And he always emptied the chamber pot just before the breakfast arrived. Although the bed was the matrimonial space where he first imagined me, my mother had been relegated to another room at the other end of the landing.

In my late teens when I had discovered some intimacy with women, I wondered how exactly he had managed to woo her, or where and when and how they had managed to copulate, but I could never get my head around the formulation of precise images.

I know he returned to work in the afternoon on the sixth of August 1953, just an hour before I was born in the upstairs bedroom, so my mother must have been drained as she waddled around the kitchen preparing his dinner on that day. And from her lonely and broken reflections years later, I know she resented how quickly after the delivery she was expected to resume her duties of cooking, cleaning and generally servicing his needs.

But it is the act of copulation that I cannot contemplate. Although I know that in his last years – the years of the blue suit – she seemed to fall in love with him for the first time. They spent their days together. She sat on the bed in the morning looking out the window, chattering about the neighbours and the small adventures of the coming day; her attendance at ten o'clock mass and who she might meet was always on the agenda, and his duties as honorary secretary of the National Council for the Blind, Cavan branch, an office of which he was extremely proud, got extensive analysis.

I could hear their mumbling voices at all hours of the day and night because even though they had an empty nest by then and my brother and I were gone to college, I did go home regularly and sleep in the small bedroom I was born in and listen at night to their voices in the next room chatting and sometimes laughing. One day I caught them in the kitchen holding an embrace which they seemed embarrassed about the moment I opened the door.

She even shared stories with me about his courage when they were young. He was in the St Vincent de Paul as secretary, she said, and at one meeting he spoke up for a family who were destitute and ought to be given money from the charity. The chairman of the committee was the manager of a local factory where the destitute man in question happened to be involved in a strike, and so the chairman blocked my father's proposal.

And my father resigned.

'That was the kind of man your father was,' my mother would say.

There was another story about her wedding that she recounted regularly.

She had wanted a particular priest who was a friend of her family to officiate at the ceremony, but the local clergy said no; only weddings conducted by the resident clerics could be allowed in the cathedral. And the cathedral was a prestigious venue. But my mother really wanted the family friend to be involved, so my father stood his ground, and they were married, to the infuriation of the local priest, not in the cathedral but outside the town in the small and beautiful church of Killygarry.

And I could only conclude that there were other stories and other issues involved which caused him to keep clerics as much as he could outside the front door.

If there was something in him that she clung to through all the years of their flawed marriage it was his integrity. When he died after a long-drawn-out illness at the age of seventy-three she was so devastated and broken that she never quite recovered from the trauma.

If he had lived longer, he might have told me more as I grew older. Who knows, he might have taken pen to paper and written a memoir and unburdened himself of all his secrets, failures and the small intimacies that make a mediocre life magnificent.

As I walked on that final trek of twenty-six kilometres I kept imagining what he might say to me now. I had already shaped an image of him: frightened and secretive. But if I had been older, would he have explained more? For in a sense he told me nothing and all I knew was what I conjectured on the long road to Santiago.

Maybe it was poetry they spoke of, him and my mother in old age. Maybe it was faith. Maybe he shared the secrets of his grandmother's origins, where she came from and what his life had been like as a child or what terrible conditions he had experienced that caused him to be so emotionally crippled as an adult.

Those secrets he took to the grave with him. Nor did she in her old age let him down by revealing anything further about his background or their love life. Perhaps there was no love life to talk about. Or perhaps she had just forgotten.

I was more than tired on that last day. I was exhausted. And with fatigue comes emotional troughs. I began to wonder if it was wise to have dwelled so long with his memory, to the extent that he was walking beside me and my mother too seemed close enough that I might reach out and touch her.

And sometimes it doesn't feel right to go picking over the past, when people are long gone.

But when both parents have died there is a portal that closes on the past and the child must move on; whatever secrets the past contained are lost forever. Or ought to be. The ghosts can no longer be permitted to attend us. Their unresolved stories are meaningless. The universe they once inhabited no longer exists. We must let go of them, otherwise we are doomed to carry them as our burden through life and ultimately to our own graves.

I certainly didn't want to do that with my parents. My pilgrimage was turning into an exorcism.

To bid him farewell.

I remember him trying to play with the child I was, but he was useless. Even at six I could see he was affecting the posture of a footballer. He wasn't really a man who had the slightest interest in kicking balls around the lawn. Although he was slightly better with a croquet set, an exotic game of heavy balls and hoops that stuck in the ground and through which the player was required to hit the balls with a long mallet. He joked on one occasion that it was like polo without the horses. But what, I wondered, was polo.

At least the elaborate lawn game was almost enjoyable for half an hour and familiarity with it built affection, as is the way in childhood, so that eventually I could pass a quiet afternoon on the lawn with the balls, the hoops and the sound of clacking mallets as I played against myself and talked to Dominic Savio, a saint and casual acquaintance who lived behind the garden hedge.

It was only when I went to college and met boys who had spent their adolescence sweating on football pitches that I realised my childhood had been so lonely.

And when the time came for me to play games with my own daughter on the lawn in summertime I found him there again. A trans-generational lack of playfulness. My failure to kick balls or swat tennis rackets or even hide and seek were disabilities in me that burned with his presence. What I lacked was like an empty space where I found him again and again. Unless of course I tried to introduce croquet to the sloping lawns of Leitrim, but that would have been a foolish endeavour considering the rushes and soggy soil.

And since he rarely frequented public houses, I found it curious that it was there especially that I thought I could find him. Not that there was anything but random coincidences governing my youth and my years in Glangevlin. It just so happened that I was sheltering there under a bawdy, robust mantle of masculinity when he died. I found in public houses the mythic energy of men that he could never guide me to. Just like the bar in Cork where I discovered that there were real writers in the world, though he was not among them.

For fifty years I dragged him around, barely conscious of the weight on my heart, or his propensity to drag me into melancholy. He was a heavy burden in so far as I only felt emptiness when he came to mind.

It's a strange thing to say, that your father was an empty space, but that's the sensation I had coming to the end of my pilgrimage. He passed to me this empty cavity of the heart, this longing without an object.

And ever since I have clung to elders, and priests, and even God with an unsatisfied longing. It was not just in the bars that he was a ghostly presence, where scholars and poets in linen suits performed, but even alone on the road to Santiago, when I ought to be fired up with the impending completion of my Camino, or the zeal of a devout pilgrim. I was empty. I was tired of him and his haunting presence.

So, I just stopped thinking about him. I absorbed the sound of booted feet before me and behind me and the birds in trees above me and the sound of traffic racing on the highway towards Santiago in the distance and it felt good to be empty.

Conjecturing about his life was a waste of time. He was an empty shell. There was nothing in him.

But there was nothing in me either. Maybe that was the gift he left me.

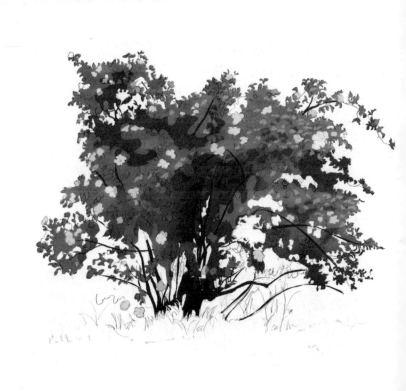

The Teacher

I had recovered from the night of shame, breakfasted alone, dawdled through town and lingered at the church on the outskirts where I saw the blind man and his daughter. But by midmorning Santiago was still eighteen kilometres away and the thunderclouds gathered and threatened to explode. The sky darkened, turned purple and with crash and blaze the rain fell, leaving all of us on the pathway scrambling to don our plastic cloaks and anoraks and jackets. Everyone got soaked, as we plodded through what in half an hour turned to stretches of muddy pathway.

The trail led through a jungle of forest, woodland and along the banks of roaring rivers with miles of slippery muck. My swanky but light anorak was useless because it wasn't waterproof, a detail I never checked in the shop when I bought it, and I got drenched to the skin.

After about ten kilometres I stopped for a coffee at a wayside restaurant and found myself sitting beside the elderly Dubliner whom I had seen in the breakfast room that morning.

He was enjoying a pot of tea and a croissant so enticing that I ordered the same and asked did he mind if I sat beside him.

He was older than me by about ten years and much wetter, but extremely cheerful.

'Do you not mind the rain?' I asked.

'It's wonderful,' he said. 'It will keep the day cool for the rest of the walk.'

Around us young people with rucksacks and walking sticks were sharing apples, peeling bananas, munching chocolate bars and plastering their blistered feet.

'Aren't the young ones great!' he declared.

'What age are you?' I wondered.

'I am eighty,' he replied.

'And why are you walking the Camino?'

'No reason,' he replied. 'But I like the young people; they're lovely.'

I'm sure he had other reasons for walking but he wasn't telling me. Instead, we spoke of public transport and driving cars in Dublin and the importance of cats in human flourishing. He was witty and bright and radiated a sense of faith. He seemed happy, as if life had been good to him. His wife was at home, he said, his children lived around the world, and he had grandchildren everywhere.

Yet he was walking through the muddy forests of Galicia alone, just to feel he was part of a tribe.

'That's what young people do for us old folk,' he said. 'They give us hope.'

Then he stared at my trousers, sizing me up from toe to head. My wet anorak was lying on the seat beside me.

'Are those the trousers you've been walking in all week?' he wondered. A rhetorical question to underline his astonishment.

'Yes,' I said, 'they're the trousers of a suit.'

'A suit?' he screamed. 'Are you mad?'

'No.'

'Where's the rest of it?'

'It's in the rucksack,' I said, and I got out the little bundle and unfurled the top of a beautiful double-breasted suit.

Returning his gaze to the trousers, which were soaking wet, he just said, 'Why?'

'Well, these trousers turned out to be very useful,' I explained. 'They're 85 per cent wool and 15 per cent silk. And for some reason extremely cool when the sun is shining.'

'And what about now in this deluge?' he asked.

'Well, to be honest,' I said, 'the material doesn't stick to my legs and they dry very quickly. So they're perfect.'

'But it's a suit,' he declared, still horrified. 'You're walking the Camino in a double-breasted suit. You're mad.'

I had enjoyed the suit all along. In the evenings I used to put on the jacket when I was going down for an evening meal in any hotel and I felt appropriately dressed, rather than in the shorts and boots and T-shirts that were common in the dining area among the men.

'You're wearing a suit on the Camino,' he repeated, as horrified as if I had been naked. 'Are you mad or what?' he repeated. 'That suit must have cost a fortune.'

'But that's where you're wrong,' I chirped. 'It cost me fifteen euro in a charity shop.'

We were bantering as men do. Slagging each other. Having a friendly bit of fun by poking at the other's image. He finished his croissant and was using the dregs of his tea to swallow a few tablets he took from a vial in his breast pocket.

'Oh,' I declared, 'I see you're not a well man.'

'Don't worry,' he retorted, 'your time will come.'

I laughed and said, 'I may be only seventy but I'm right there with you already.' And I held aloft my own supply of little white pills in a yellow vial that was divided into seven days of the week.

I dropped five into my palm and, like him, swallowed them with the dregs of my tea.

'Bisoprolol, candesartan, aspirin,' I intoned. 'Actase, vitamin D.'

'What's wrong with you?'

I laughed. Where could I begin?

Such encounters are common on the Camino walk. You have a casual conversation with someone, and a tiny thread of connectivity is established over a coffee or soup. You bid them farewell and begin walking again, and by chance in some *albergue* later in the day you see them again sitting alone in a corner. So you go over and share a coffee, and pick up the talk where you left off hours earlier.

And by the following morning you are both walking, not together but in a kind of unison, bumping into each other casually at the restaurants along the route and picking up the conversation from each previous meeting.

'Do you have things that go through your mind as you're walking?' I wondered.

'No,' he said. 'I'm just . . . empty. It's the best way.'

I could have said, *Thank you, my teacher*. But I didn't. I just said, 'Me too. The walk empties the mind. That's it. You've said it perfectly.'

This stranger was almost a decade older than my father when he died. And yet he was alive and humorous, and robustly healthy for his years, and I loved him for that. There was a lightness about our conversation almost akin to intimacy which buoyed me up with energy for the remaining walk.

We gathered up our wet gear and looked grimly at the sky, clutched our walking sticks and went back to the road; him to his path and I to mine.

Empty.

And I lost sight of him.

He vanished into the crowd ahead of me. Though I had a suspicion he'd turn up again somewhere. After all, we were both heading towards the same destination.

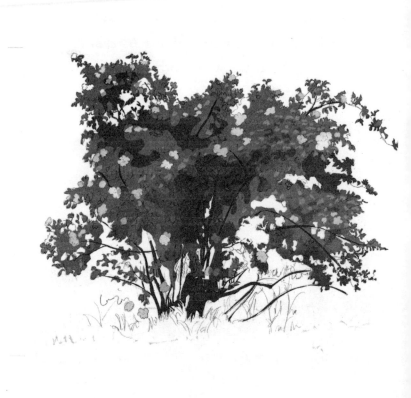

The Writer

I walked a very long time that afternoon in rain. Longer than I had ever imagined I'd be able to when I left hospital in 2021. I had come to walk with my father and figure out who exactly he was. I wanted to focus on the lacuna he left in me, the absence I could never understand. And all of it was founded on the premise that I did not know my father. That there was something there to know.

Yet suddenly in the middle of a casual exchange with a stranger, something got said that lifted me up.

Maybe there wasn't anything there to know. Maybe life is incomplete, contingent on random events and gathers around no authentic self. Maybe the I in me is merely a delusion. Maybe the I in my father never existed. Being here may be just the surface of something that is not I but thou, in the reverential phrase of Martin Buber contemplating the cosmos.

And that was his gift to me. Like the old Dubliner, he was empty when he walked.

And there I was for days gathering up images of my father from the past like I might be stuffing old pound notes in a jam jar for safe-keeping; as if they were valuable. When all the time I ought to have been divesting my mind of dross, of memories and emotion and just walking on.

And maybe there is nothing in any of us. Maybe there is no essential self and no need to hug it and nurse it and worry about it. Maybe we are all empty.

Perhaps I shared more with my father than I had realised. Perhaps he too was a teacher of wisdom and resigned in his later years to just sit in an armchair, or lie on a deckchair in the back garden beside the rose bush with a handkerchief stretched across his forehead to protect himself from the sun. Maybe he understood there was nothing more to grasp. Nothing to worry about in the emptiness of being. Leave it all to the angels.

As a teenager I wrote a poem about the future.

> Someday I'll go to the city and look at
> the filth and the dirt
> And I'll roll around in it, because poets
> are a dirty lot
> And my jeans will be faded, my hair in a
> mess
> And I'll write of death and decaying
> matter
> And how I had an unhappy childhood.
> And all will say, the boy has talent
> Because he lives like a beggar
> And writes what he shouldn't.
> But I wish I could stay at home in the
> field
> With the lake and the trees and the sun
> going down
> And the thought of a day that I've just
> put behind me and the thought of
> another that's coming my way.

I posted it to David Marcus, literary editor of *The Irish Press*. I was sixteen. Within a week I received a reply. It sat on the dining-room table all day while I was at school. I came home on the bus, worrying about Leaving Cert honours maths classes, which I had recently begun. I had completed the Inter Cert and was being forced to do honours maths against my will.

I loved history and English, but maths frightened me. I feared the following two years might likely shatter my self-confidence and destroy any sense of worth I was developing. Instead of allowing me to do subjects I loved and write poetry, I was informed that my future was in numbers which I hadn't any possibility of comprehending.

In those days I studied in an empty dining room, at a sombre mahogany table, on which the letter had been left by my father unopened.

The table was bought in a swanky store in Dublin where my father had once worked as a child, packing boxes. Because he was obliged to sell newspapers on the streets every afternoon to help support his family, he missed the end of each school day and it so happened that the final lesson in those days was algebra. So, like other poor children, he never got beyond adding and subtracting.

Being cheated out of what he loved, the magic of numbers, he resolved to make them part of his adult life. When he lost his job packing boxes at Pim's on George's Street, due to the onset of an economic depression, he decided to change his life and begin night classes. And there began the long apprenticeship of menial jobs by day and correspondence courses by night, from Rathmines to the University of Glasgow, until he eventually reached the dizzy heights of a profession, and became county accountant for Cavan.

Married in his fifties, he went back to an old friend who had packed boxes with him as a child and bought a sideboard, four chairs and the dining-room table at which I did my homework.

I loved that table. I saw it as a symbol of my father's journey and struggle, and when my parents were long dead and the old house was being sold I made sure to take the table with me to Leitrim where I intended it to function as a temporary addition to our humble abode until we got furniture of our own. But it lasted the length of my own child's childhood, and I would come home sometimes and smile to find her sitting there in the evenings attending to whatever absorbed her on the screen of her laptop.

Antique furniture is never immediate in its affective power. Old mahogany is replete with nostalgia: the hand-carved tabletops, the curved lines, the fluted legs and arms resonate with the echo of ghosts and souls long gone from the earth. All these works of art in dark wood are the remnants of lives already finished and even the people who commissioned the furniture and wrote epistles at those writing desks and sofa tables are all in their graves.

Antique furniture surrounds me with a soft nostalgia for times past, the impermanence of history, as it folds me in a blanket of solitude, like when one is awake in the night and all others in the house are in their beds asleep. Thus sleep the dead that once crafted the chair I sit on and the Maple & Co. partner desk on which I write my own chronicle of passing time.

The parlour room above the bar in Castlepollard may have been my first writer's studio, my first monastic cell, where I woke in the lattice of yellow light streaming through the lace curtains and discovered myself astride two worlds: that which was on the outside and trembled with life, and that which was within, as opaque as moonlight in an empty sky. On the outside, the world was stuffed with real people hammering on with their cares and woes. But on the inside, there was only the stillness of being. Maybe that was really my father's ghost.

Even in my early thirties I clung to the faded grandeur of those old parlour rooms, the antique furniture and the nostalgic light that poured from dim lamps on Victorian mantelpieces, and I sought out such places that were old and refined and which gave me comfort. None better or more comforting than the small back lounge in the Clarence Hotel where in the 1980s a famous sports journalist often passed his time, in denim working trousers that a man might wear in a farmyard, and a grey shapeless T-shirt hanging loosely on his enormous frame, while his grey hair fell almost to his shoulders. A whale of a man striding in slow motion across the green carpet of that tiny lounge, looking so anxious that he might have been the Christ, Yeshua, if Yeshua had been relieved from the agony of his crucifixion and gone on to survive somewhere hidden in the cafés and bazaars of Arabia. Although I expect Yeshua might have drunk a lot of coffee in the afternoon shade to cope with his trauma.

Physically he was most unlike my father and yet in him too I found fatherhood. It was like being close to a feral animal who protects you. Houlihan was an elderly lion. And it's what I longed for. His voice was a heartbroken whisper, full of the clarity of compassion when he spoke of Kerry footballers or the people who loved them.

He was shy and spoke with reticence, his face hidden by an enormous hand covering his mouth and eyes, as if the light of something before him was enough to blind him.

He would come over to me and make observations on the mystery of life. He would praise me for one play I had written and which he had seen at the Abbey Theatre. He would tell me over again each time how it reminded him of his childhood in Kerry. It was the liturgy of our meeting. My Yeshua came with the same words of welcome each time.

'You wrote something wonderful,' he would begin.

Then he'd sit and say nothing for a long while, as I spluttered out my confused notions about the meaning of life. And after five or ten minutes he'd smile and go to the bar, a little stall in the centre of the dark lounge, order himself another drink and forget to come back to my corner.

His vulnerability was beautiful and for a time my own dark stranger within dissolved into this benign creature, my father became incarnate in the lion before me, and I dared to hope that after a few more decades I might be moulded into such an heroic embodiment of woundedness.

I am old now and like all old people I could say that I wander in a strange land without direction. I could say too that Con was there before me, walking the path before me, and possessing the maps without ever saying an explicit word. That's what I think fathers do in the end.

They know the emptiness and the lightness of the empty mind, and they reassure their children not by what they say but by what they embody.

They are a presence.

And eventually a person sees that the old feeble one with white spindled legs called Daddy is just a facade; the walking stick and breathlessness are a role played out in a moment of time. Suit or hospital gown, it's just another costume for another performance and another role.

But if you look with the heart, you see the lion. The being behind the empty shell. And you begin to see the father in all old men whose ways are gentle. Which is what I had not noticed, when my own little daddy was clutching the cot sides of the bed he died in. Like I was still too young to realise that I ought to have been searching for the lion, and not the old man.

The letter that lay unopened long ago in my youth was addressed to me in bold type, which indicated that it must be from an adult. And there was only one adult who might be writing to me in such an officious tone, using a white business-class envelope and affixing the title Esquire to the end of my name.

I didn't open it instantly. I needed to get my maths homework out of the way. If I opened the envelope and read a letter of rejection before I opened my maths books, I wouldn't have been able to finish any homework.

So, I slipped the letter between the pages of Patrick Kavanagh's collected works which had been published about a year earlier and which was to me a sacred text during those days.

Eventually before bedtime I opened and read the parchment written and signed by David Marcus.

It was like reading something from Moses. Like listening to the verdict of a remote judge. The editor-in-chief of the most important poetry platform in the nation was addressing me. And he liked the poems. And he wanted to publish them.

In those days I used to get the bus to school, but I might as well have been a ghost. Neither the Loreto girls in their burgundy skirts nor the demure daughters of the Royal School ever bothered with me. I didn't play football, didn't have long hair and was never in trouble with the police; so, I was a complete non-entity.

Getting in trouble with various police forces would have been easy in those days even if I was only sixteen. In Enniskillen, where we went regularly as a family to buy butter, there were always RUC men patrolling the street outside Woolworths, fingering their pistols as they glared at young boys like me, and I'm sure the slightest impudence would have brought their ire down upon me as I brushed past them in search of Milky Way bars that were not available in the Free State.

Non-entities like me dreamed of such drama. How wonderful it would have been if the story got out in Loreto that I was in trouble with the RUC.

It never happened. Although it wasn't the RUC that I feared. It was my mother who policed my adolescence as if I were a medieval prince. She marked out the social boundaries I dared not cross. And being rude with uniformed officers in Enniskillen was the gravest of boundaries; particularly since our car was stuffed with so much butter on the way home.

I was so incompetent at everything that I couldn't even get arrested for not having a light on my bicycle. And I did try regularly, but without success.

There was a guard in Cavan at the time who was zealous about the law regarding bicycle lamps. He would wait in the bushes or behind a low wall of suburbia, watching for college students cycling home after official study hours at night, hoping to catch someone who wasn't adequately illuminated. Even my mother thought he was an ignoramus, so it was a notoriety I could have aspired to without fearing her wrath if I had ended up in court. I regularly cycled out in front of the pack, alone and as visible as a black cat in a coal shed, but I was never fortunate enough to do it on a night when the guard was on duty.

It would have been an heroic narrative had I been caught, and might have secured me more attention on the school bus, but at sixteen I had resigned myself to a life of invisibility.

Then the poems were published, and my life changed.

The Beatles had recorded a few LPs and Bob Dylan whined and wailed on transistor radio sets beneath the pillows of a thousand young girls all over the country, and some of them sat by day on my school bus, and up until then, if ever I brushed past their shoulders they remained as detached as zen monks.

But being a poet trumped even playing football. An heroic figure, solitary and melancholic, languishing in an attic and writing love poems, would have been a matchless prize for any girl in burgundy or green. And sure enough the moment I stepped onto the dance floor in Cavan after that first publication I realised I had become a different person. At teenage dances, or 'hops' as we used to call them, I slung my coat over my shoulders like it were a Yeatsian cloak and for eighteen more months I strode along the aisle of the school bus like a great colossus of wounded grace.

I never mentioned this aspect of my good fortune to David Marcus when I met him for the first time some years later in his home in Dublin. Even then I was terrified of adults who had achieved so much in life.

But I remember him being curious about my life as a writer and so I mumbled to him something

I LOVED HIM FROM THE DAY HE DIED

about a book I was working on and how I hoped it would be published.

'Oh, it will,' he said with assurance, 'it will.' And then he added, 'The first of many, I hope.'

For me that moment was as life-altering as the first letter, though it was just a casual remark. In that one supportive phrase my self-image was reframed again. He was graciously presuming that I might be on a pathway as a writer for the long-term.

David Marcus influenced the shape of my life in both those moments. Brief and terse and casual, yet transformative for me. I felt his presence constantly as a mentor and teacher to whom I remained deeply indebted.

There were further letters from Mr Marcus, and further poems by me in *The Irish Press*. There were short stories too, and some years later I received a Hennessy Award, which was another milestone on the way towards life as a full-time writer.

It was David Marcus who advised me to use the title Michael P. Harding on my first book, since my father was already known as Michael Harding from his regular book reviews in the same news-paper.

All my opportunities for writing and publishing were direct or indirect consequences of that first letter, and of David Marcus's confidence in my writing, and the generosity with which he treated me as a writer as if he were sure that I had a future.

And my father was quietly proud. Even though I may have written an occasional disparaging line about my childhood or my relationship with him, he never flinched in the face of poetry. Whenever he saw me at that old table in the dining room opening other letters or reading anything other than schoolbooks he would say, 'I won't interrupt you, you're at your work.'

And I don't think it was a casual remark. After all, he had strong opinions about education and was clear enough on numerous occasions about my initial year spent in a seminary. Yet when it came to poetry and writing, he always peered over my shoulder and whispered, 'Keep it up.'

My father died only seven years after those first poems were published, and the table outlasted him by almost fifty years. Then one leg collapsed and the tabletop was recycled as a work bench in the garden shed. It even outlasted David Marcus by almost fifteen years. It was a good table.

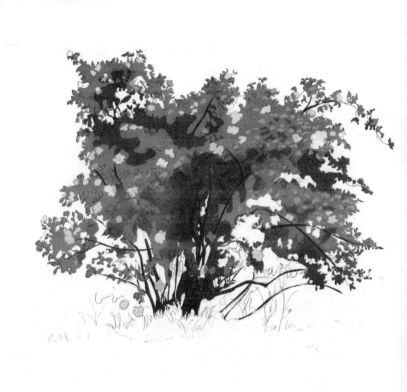

Cloisters of the Heart

How happy I was that I asked the travel agency in Ireland to book me into the best hotel they could find for two nights when the walk was completed. I wanted a jacuzzi and sauna and a pool to swim in. I wanted five stars and a king-size bed. The suffering over, I'd be entitled to indulge myself.

Convento de San Francisco was once a medieval convent of nuns. Now it is a hotel of quiet elegance. The shell has been retained with the inner courtyard, refectory and library. The rest is glass and metal girders, tastefully opening up an interior of ghosts from Catholic Spain.

The refectory alone is arranged as it always was in medieval days, with the seating for monks around the walls intact, the high ceilings echoing with voices of monastic choirs from hidden speakers, and the gable end of the space is dressed with images and icons illustrating the life and death of the most remarkable Judean teacher and storyteller the world has ever seen. Yeshua, as they call him nowadays.

'Jesus Christ,' I muttered at reception, 'I'm fucking drenched to the skin.'

I don't think the concierge was impressed. She just winced.

My suitcase as usual had been taken from hotel to hotel and the lady at reception said it was already in my room. She gave me the key, told me the room number and wished me a pleasant stay. My yellow backpack was dripping, so I asked her if it would be okay to take a little walk around before I went upstairs, and she smiled through her teeth and said of course. But I don't think she had recovered from my vain use of the holy name.

I went down the cloister and into the great refectory and stared in awe at the red velvet seating, the high ceiling, the images of Christ and his Mother, and I was thinking this is the best fucking hotel I've ever been in. It didn't feel like a hotel at all. It retained the austere and contemplative air of a convent.

And when I was walking back through the cloister who did I see sitting on a bench in pensive mood but the old man from Dublin, with his long silver hair well combed into a ponytail at the back of his head, and no trace of the long weary march in his face. He was wearing the same clothes as on the road but no sign of boots, rucksack or rain gear. The sandals wrapped around his bony feet gave him the air of someone who might have been sitting there for centuries, just like the statues of St Francis and other monks that adorned the corridors.

'I got a taxi,' he confessed. 'Twenty-six kilometres was too much for me. I did about fifteen and then they picked me up.'

Neither of us was surprised by this meeting. We had both booked with U Walk and naturally they use the same hotels and *albergues* along the route for all their pilgrims.

'We must meet later,' I suggested, and he agreed. So, I left him in contemplation on the cloister and went to my room. I noted how fragile his body was at more than eighty years of age. Something

I had not noticed earlier because the lion in him was so strong.

St James as mentioned in the Gospels was another lion, and perhaps a sibling of Yeshua himself. It's a long story or a good yarn as to how he ended up in Galicia, but in any event, the city of Santiago is a powerful stone citadel on a hill and the name translates as St James. And Compostela according to more stories might mean 'a field of stars'. Although some say it means 'a burial ground'.

But I never realised how mystical the city of Santiago de Compostela could be, or why so many would want to walk from the ends of the earth to get there. I had brazened it with a light rucksack and taken the lazy route, walking 120 kilometres over ten days rather than five. And my room in the convent hotel was a bastion of silence, and I slept like a baby, with all the garish saints of ancient times in their sumptuous costumes and vestments, holding their swords and sticks and staffs, glaring sometimes from behind altars at me in my dreams.

I never envy young people who take photos of these saints with their smartphones, nonchalantly passing from one altar to the next and taking selfies before high altars, because young people must live on the surface in order to respond to the sensate invitations that construct the cosmos in which they are called to become. It's what human birth is all about; we are flung onto the surface of reality and it takes us a lifetime to find its hidden depth. It's only in old age that the plaster statues and garish saints become clear to us.

The following day was Sunday so I went to the cathedral, where crowds were queuing at the door. Once inside I found space in a pew next to a Spanish woman with outstretched hands as she gazed up at the figure of St James above the altar with her two eyes closed. The rest of the pilgrims were settling in the pews before the midday mass and using their phones to capture the magnificent architecture. Many of them were kitted out in hiking boots with water bottles dangling from rucksacks. The lady beside me calmed down and the mass began and the sermon was in Spanish, and we stood and knelt at different times for various prayers, and when the priest intoned the words *pax Dominum vobiscum*, I turned to her and expected to receive her hand in a formal greeting of peace, but instead she put her arms around me and clasped me fiercely like her son. I reciprocated and felt as relaxed as if I had just embraced my mother.

There's a square to the side of the cathedral with various open-air cafés where people eat and drink. She sat alone at a table after mass and caught my eye, so I went over to say hello. She spoke English and I managed to exchange a few words with her.

'Did you see the moon?' she asked me.

'No,' I replied. 'I didn't notice.'

'But there was a full moon last night,' she said. 'You must see it. It will open your heart.'

I hadn't seen the moon on my walking days, probably because at night I was too exhausted to look out the window, but in fact the full moon was promised that weekend.

'I will see it tonight,' I said to her.

'Of course,' she agreed. 'It will be the same moon tonight.'

She meant that it would still be a full moon that night but I was thinking of what Rumi said; that the soul is like a mirror, reflecting the divine presence; just like a lake reflects the moon.

'Yes,' I agreed. 'It will be the same moon tonight.'

For me the moon has always been magical and always the same, whether in Glangevlin or Santiago. It transports me into a different realm. It is the one and only moon I have. The same and only moon that shines on the streets of Paris or in the deserts of Mongolia. The same moon I saw so many years ago at the Shannon Pot, and that shimmered on the surface of a certain lake in Galilee where James the apostle went fishing with his brothers. The same moon that Islamic scholars across Spain might have seen when they quenched their candles late in the night and gazed out from their towers.

And although I have spent my life in the shadow of various cathedrals and prayer halls, it is the moon above that kept me company in the dark. As my father did, in all the crowded spaces of the day and on every kilometre of the journey.

I was hoping to have a swim because the hotel had a pool in a separate building in the back garden. And nobody used it. I had looked in the previous evening and it was empty. And again on Sunday morning before I went to mass, I checked and again it was empty.

So after mass I got a towel from reception, and a key for a locker, and went to the pool.

Completely empty. I had the place to myself. The pool was still, the surface like glass, and it reminded me of a text in the Gospel, where Jesus comes to the pool of Bethsaida. The invalids are waiting on stretchers. And the story is that sometimes an angel will descend and touch the waters and then whoever gets in first to the pool will be healed. But one guy can't walk so he can never get to the water. Jesus listens to him as he explains, and then Jesus says, 'Take up your bed and be healed.'

And the man is made whole again.

Wisdom in the Gospels is wrapped in stories. They are like koans or Sufi yarns. They draw me in and allow me to walk around inside them without ever making logical sense. And whenever I finish reading a little story from the Gospel I feel I've heard Jesus the storyteller, the Sufi teacher. I suppose the Gospels are opaque enough to appeal to everyone in different ways. And I'm a storyteller, so what's so surprising that I see Yeshua as a storyteller too?

I was in the jacuzzi which overlooks the still surface of the swimming pool, drenched in sunlight from floor-to-ceiling windows.

And then I heard a noise. Another guest arriving; a man in the changing compartment. I heard him shuffle off his clothes before he emerged through the door. Wearing only a swim cap and black shorts, it took me a moment to realise it was my friend from Dublin.

He went to the little ladder that draws the swimmer into the pool. He dipped his toe through the glass surface of the water. He descended. The water cracked and rippled as he leaned into it and began to swim ever so slowly to the far end of the pool.

Fuck this, I thought, frustrated that my glorious solitude had been disturbed.

But then I noticed that he had stopped at the far end. He was holding the ladder and stood rubbing his face, or perhaps his eyes. I thought for a moment some dirt or water or chlorine had irritated him. But then I realised he was weeping. I imagined half a dozen reasons why this might be so. I speculated about what family he might have, or what bereavement he had not mentioned. There was an unlimited amount of possibilities. But he was not aware that I had noticed him. In fact I don't think he saw me there at all. And the moment passed and he began swimming again.

I left the jacuzzi, got dressed and went away. The saddest thing about men is that they cry alone. It's not a failure. It is just sometimes a man understands his own solitude and is sorrowful. And sometimes it is gratitude that brings a man to tears. And when I saw the full moon over Santiago that night from my hotel window, I knew that if there was a moment for me to cry it was exactly then.

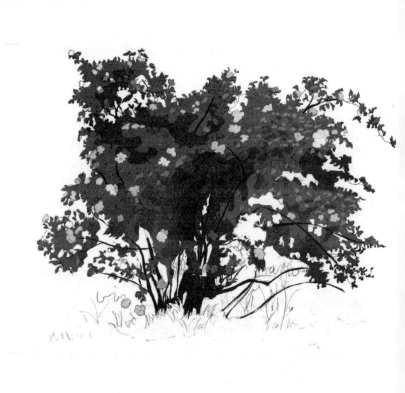

The Roses

Just over a week after my father died, I was spending the eve of my twenty-third birthday in the sunshine in the back garden of the house in Cavan where I had grown up, staring at the rose bushes that were no longer in bloom.

Those roses meant nothing to me in childhood. I often crashed the push-mower into the base when I was mowing the lawn, scattering showers of pale pink petals onto the grass. It didn't bother me to abuse them. They were just one more obstacle among many that I had to negotiate with the lawnmower to keep the grass low.

But after the death I sat there in early August staring at them and at the dying petals on the grass wondering why he planted them. It was a pink rose. Like crimson blood seeping into a white bandage, it was a watery pale-pink petal.

They had begun their life in County Clare. My father replanted them in Cavan behind the house which had just been built for him and his new wife. It was one of those rare and uncharacteristically romantic gestures he was sometimes capable of. And it's not even something he spoke about with any enthusiasm. In fact, based on what he said when I was growing up, he might not have known the roses were there at all.

It was my mother who said it, often.

'Your father brought those roses from Clare,' she would say, suggesting that she remembered the moment with more affection than he did.

I imagine them in their little flat in the middle of Cavan town, having discussions with the seller of the land, and then with the builder, and maybe walking out from town in the evenings to witness the ongoing work of digging foundations, raising walls and framing the wooden roof. The house was a semi-detached building and one of a pair situated on a hill side by side beyond the town boundary.

On their honeymoon, for which they retained

an album of photographs and postcards, they journeyed from the Bush Hotel in Carrick-on-Shannon as far south as Kerry, stopping in Ennis on the way. That's as much as the postcards in the wedding album could tell me. Although my imagination often filled in the rest.

It's likely they would have visited the woman who presided over the boarding house where he had lodged in the late forties, just before he came to Cavan and met her.

I'm sure the elderly Mrs Davoren would have loved to meet his new bride. Maybe that's when Mrs Davoren said he should have a couple of plants as a wedding gift. Maybe she had noted over the years when he lived there that he lingered close to them in the garden on summer evenings. Maybe the gesture, the roses, the romantic moment was something my mother was caught up in, and said yes, and so the roses ended up in the car, hired from Flood's of Bridge Street for the occasion of the honeymoon. And perhaps it reflects on the hardness of his heart that she remembered those roses often as she gazed out the window, while he forgot.

What was he feeling when he lifted those tiny shrubs from the garden in Ennis and brought them to adorn the back garden of his new home?

Did he imagine himself in old age sitting where I was sitting, admiring them? Did it hurt him when I ploughed into them with the push lawn-mower because I was a teenager and didn't give a fuck what old people felt or thought? That's where my obsession with the roses began.

My father was a bloodless man, as far as I could tell by looking at him. And I saw him naked often enough in his last few years as he lay sometimes all summer long between the cot sides of a hospital bed where due to medical neglect he developed enormous bed sores on his hips. They were open wounds. I looked one day and saw what I presumed was the white knuckle of his hip and the juicy white flesh with a pink hue as the nurse dressed it with ointments and disinfectant cream and white gauze.

The nurse said I could leave the room while she was working, but I shrugged off the suggestion and remained in my chair, legs crossed, hands folded, trying not to scream for poor Daddy, as the old man in the bed groaned and the nurse repeated her best soothing line: 'I'm nearly finished.'

The sun went down and the back garden sank into shadow and I went into the house to spend the remains of the day watching television alone.

I stayed in Cavan that night but my mother was away mourning with her sister in Castlepollard. I slept in the big double bed, which felt like drowning in the place where he first imagined me. I felt tethered to him for life.

I was angry with him because I might have wished to spend the night in his company. Instead the only thing I could do was absorb the shadowy silence of the house and grab some memories of him and store them for the future.

I was vulnerable that night, like a child with a lantern in the wind and no hand on my shoulder to guide me. How could I fend for myself without a real father?

I recoiled at the memory of his body in the last months of his life. I was angry with him for having withered. I hated to think I would end up like him. I clenched my fists and closed my eyes as if I was a rock being battered with the flung spray of the ocean. My fragility was his fault. He was the shade that begot me. And now he was the demon that was eating me alive.

I wanted to be a priest but he didn't approve. I wanted to be a success but he was a poor role model to be saddled with. I would have settled for being anything but his son. Not that I wished to be unborn, but just not his son.

My mother had lightened my childhood with confessions about how she wished her second child had been a girl. But she was disappointed.

I wondered if being a daughter might have been different. It might have put a distance between us. I could have laid claim to an alternative universe; a world of tenderness and intimacy as opposed to the stale masculinity of his old withered carcass.

Yet it was in masculinity I was born, and some part of me still cried out to him with love. Even his sour and broken body was beautiful and elegant in its decay. I felt like a man when I shouldered his coffin, and as his coffin was lowered into the ground some part of his soul was beginning to flourish in me. I saw him in the mirror in the bedroom that night and his presence was still burning in me, even beyond his death, and I loved him as a son.

So early the following morning I bent over the old mahogany table in the dining room and wrote a poem to mark the closure of his life and the beginning of my love, before I left the house.

I posted it a few days later to David Marcus and hoped to see it published in the paper later in the autumn.

The House in August
(In Memoriam)

The day you died I stuffed images
Like old pound notes in a jam jar.
My hooked eyes were full of promises.
My body a lantern
Holding its useless light
Against the dark.

Sleeping in the huge double bed
Is like drowning
In the place where you first
Imagined me.

The knuckles of my body
Closed like a rock
Against your flung spray,
Against your white sea ghosts.

Is this the way you wanted it?
The back garden still wild with weeds
Your teeth still ripping meat
From my bones?

You have hunted me away
From my own fireplace
Made me chance everything
In the dark.

I was etched on the wrong stone
A skull squeezed in a skin bag
I should have slept on a lace-edged
   pillow
I should have worn soft peach cloth
   against my shoulder
Daddy's little girl might have been
Less nervous of the dark.

In August of 1976 my mother wasn't madly fascinated with poetry, though she admired David Marcus and was proud when I told her I had more poetry being published in the newspaper. She had more to think about than just poetry: she was beginning a long life of grief without her partner, and she didn't know how to negotiate all the necessary paperwork for dissolving his existence and establishing herself as a legal widow.

I drove her to the grave in the Austin Morris 1100, a car my father purchased after the Austin A40 gave up. The Morris 1100 boasted a hydrolastic suspension system which had once been his pride and joy but which for some years had been driven only by her. Now she didn't want to drive it so I took the wheel. At the cemetery she wept and spoke to the mound of clay as if she were still talking to him in the hospital, her words barely comprehensible.

Then I drove her home and went once more to the back garden and stared at the wilting roses and the fallen petals.

Remembering my bloodless father in hospital and imagining his lifeless bones in the grave, wrapped in a suit as blue as the sky, I began to realise why lovely Yeshua the storyteller was so important to me. The crucified Christ has been for centuries a powerful icon and motif in the lexicon of meaning for human beings because it is not difficult to see human suffering in the suffering of Christ. The idea that my father's suffering contained a spiritual dimension was comforting.

Memory is an amazing thread that draws us into the weave until the entire fabric is clear. And I must record that as I sat thinking of those roses, and how my mother was the one who mentioned them, I recall that she did so at the kitchen sink, when one of them was still growing in the flower border just opposite the window.

'Your father brought those roses from Clare,' she said. It summed up all that she hoped for in that marriage. All that she was perhaps disappointed about. It was only in later years that the bush was moved, when a back kitchen was being built as an extension in place of the back yard shed.

I even remember him trying to nourish them one day after they had been moved.

My mother had a washing line that went from one side of the garden to the other, and it was draped with white sheets, well speckled with cow dung by the time my father was finished attending to the roses.

'Can you not see what you're doing?' she said with waspish irritation. And he had no reply because it was an obvious truth – he couldn't see what he was doing a lot of the time because of his bad eyes.

Twenty years after he died I moved them to the garden of the house my beloved and I had purchased in Leitrim in 1996. It wasn't my own marriage I was celebrating in the act but some bond with my father, some hope that in the ritual of the rose and in the remembrance of him, I would find an intimacy that I did not enjoy in childhood.

Though I laughed when I researched the rose and found that these five-fingered watery pink petals with big yellow stamens constituted nothing more than a weed.

A weed in Australia and New Zealand, an invasive plant in other countries, but in Leitrim a wild rose, growing on every bush and ditch, so plentiful that they had a full-blown summer festival in the county that was called the Leitrim Wild Rose Festival.

I always say we live in Leitrim, but that is because the postal address is Leitrim. Technically we live in County Roscommon, and I often point at the bushes and say that the roses may be living in Roscommon but the bees that pollinate them fly from Leitrim, because Leitrim is on three sides all around us in the next townlands.

The dog rose, the wild rose, my father's rose, whatever you call it, was mentioned in Shakespeare's play *A Midsummer Night's Dream*, and it has grown for thousands of years across the world. It was used in Poland to make a jam for doughnuts, and had roots that could cure the bite of a rabid dog, and it was often associated with the American victory in the Second World War. Yet it was a weed. The most common and humble among all the roses.

He might not have known this when he took them from Clare and then forgot about them so that only she, his wife, was left to gaze out the kitchen window for years in those moments of isolation when the bed she made turned out not to be quite the paradise she expected, and take consolation in the humble rose. Maybe that's why I stopped tending it in my own garden.

There were other roses on the patio in my own home in Leitrim. Hybrid tea roses I was trying to grow with dung provided by a neighbour who was never in an aeroplane and would always talk of far-off places when he came on his tractor in the springtime.

My beloved revealed her green mystical fingers over the years and the entire patio blossomed with colour and foliage, and I lived as content as the cats that stretched themselves in the evening sun.

The weeds were not held back, the bramble grew and rushes raised their ugly heads all around where the dog rose lived and died and was eventually forgotten.

One springtime came, and I looked out to find it but it was not there. As if some fox or dog had come and dug it out and chewed its roots away.

I planted one hundred trees to mark the milestones through the years so that in old age I might do as I do now: sit on the patio and at the towering branches that commemorate so many friends. They are all there in the summertime, flush and full of leaf and flower, dancing in the wind as I sit with a glass of wine and creaking bones. But only my father's rose is the rose that I forgot.

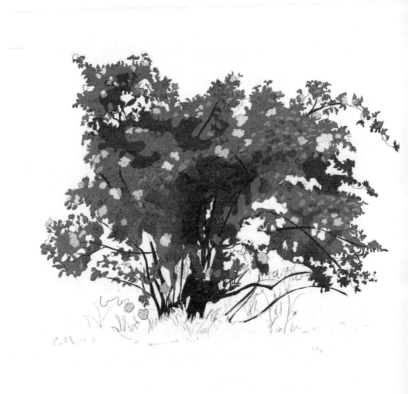

Glangevlin Adieu

Soon after I walked the Camino, I got a text message from a friend in Glangevlin saying that her mother was ill. Her mother was over eighty. And I had been to see her at Christmas, and she was her same old self, sitting on the sofa in the kitchen, beside the range, her husband sitting opposite her and her children gathered around her.

On the night I slept on the crates in Glangevlin all those years ago, Annie McGovern had been working in the mineral bar, a dark-haired woman about fifteen years my senior. I was a familiar item in her house. I would sit by the range all afternoon drinking tea, imbibing her stories and satiric humour. Glad to have her kitchen as a shelter after my father died because it was a house of love and family affection and laughter and pranks and always full of dogs. As we used to say, 'there was great fun'.

To the end she loved her dogs. When she gave up the ghost a few weeks later I returned to Glangevlin for the funeral. I drove across Glan Gap in the Cuilcagh mountains, and I stopped the car at the summit for a view of the lowlands, the plains of Fermanagh and Cavan along the rivers and Brackley lake lying like a silver coin to the east, and I walked a bit further up the mountain path that leads towards the very tip of Cuilcagh.

I remember stopping there on the mountain gap in 1971 in a little Fiat 127 on my first adventure into that beautiful world. I remember taking in a view of the valley below for the first time. A mountain wilderness that became for me a refuge, a shelter and a sacred space. Where I felt the Shannon water was holding the moon in its heart as a lover holds the beloved. And I thought of myself as water holding the reflection of a great light, like water holds the moon's reflection. The same moon. And the same beloved in every heart.

So, there I was again in Glangevlin, half a century later, for the funeral of a woman who had been such a great friend to me when she was in her late thirties, and I was in my early twenties. Annie was married with young children and sat by the range while her husband worked outside in the garage fixing tractors and cars for locals including myself; we would idle at the garage door smoking cigarettes and watch Joe the mechanic with awe, as if he were a brain surgeon, while he leaned into the engine with wrenches and a greasy face to get my Fiat 127 back on the road after it burst a gasket.

The kitchen was so close that Annie could tap the window to get his attention for a mid-morning cup of tea, and me too if I was there.

I drove cheap cars that regularly required attention, so that's how I got my feet close to the range in that wonderful kitchen of strong tea, good humour and bawdy laughter, presided over by Annie with the authority of a speaker in the houses of parliament. She would bid her German shepherd get off the sofa beside the range to make room for me.

Often a circle of neighbours sat for tea, sometimes absorbed in collective silence; everyone staring out the window or lost in their own thoughts. Because in those days conversation was not just a continuous flow of chatter. There were silences, spaces in time during which the kettle hissing on the range or the dog dreaming beneath the sofa were the only sounds to break the spell, until the talking stirred again, wit and wisdom rising from the silence like ripening fruit.

And it was that sweet silence I recalled during the funeral as the priest sat beside the altar with bowed head after communion, and grieving children sat motionless in the front pew.

Marilynne Robinson, the American novelist, says that churches are wonderful because they are the place where we make the great concession to one another that we are mortal. 'We see children baptised,' she says, 'that we will not live to see marry.'

I suppose that's what makes us capable of comforting each other. We're all in the same boat. We all look at coffins with the same unspoken fascination.

Annie knew well what Marilynne Robinson was talking about; she carried two of her children to the grave long before her own coffin was wheeled out of Glan chapel to the sound of a hymn, 'Nearer My God to Thee', played by a lonesome accordion.

And making a little procession behind the coffin were her elderly husband and her grieving children. Even the young ones, turning grey, had a lot to be silent about when the music died and only the creak of the trolly beneath the coffin could be heard in the church porch.

Someone told me that as she lay waiting for the end of life all her family gathered in the hospice. Her husband held her hand and her dearest friend, another German shepherd dog, lay on the bed beside her and watched her breathing.

The sun shone on her grave, phrases of the rosary floated on the wind, and Cuilcagh mountain above us held itself in an immense silence.

I shook her husband's strong hand as his children escorted him away but neither of us spoke. For that moment we were back again in the kitchen where the kettle sang on the range and the people who loved her gathered around to enjoy her fun and wit and laughter.

There was soup and sandwiches afterwards in the parish hall where we all used to dance on

Saturday nights, when Annie oversaw the mineral bar and dished out witty advice with every glass of lemonade or Cavan Cola that she served to the courting couples.

The sun was shining as I left the parish hall. Someone said, 'That's a lovely day now, thank God.'

And I said, 'Yes, it is. Thank God.' A casual exchange after which I just stood gazing at the valley and the sloping mountains all around me.

Maybe we all bury the dead, move on, and then find them more beautifully in a certain specific place.

In Glan I fumbled towards love and was caught up in an emotional entanglement with the hidden father that manifests in people and places we love. I laughed with farmers and bachelor poets on their broken bicycles. Glangevlin was the alcove of my heart; my cloister and my completion. I found my father there in the secret realm of love, and everything after that was merely footnotes.

I doubt if there is a sentient being born who does not have such a secret. A place in the heart where they find a capacity for love. A location secured by the heart's compass.

I see it in the cuckoo, the swallow, the winter thrush and all the other migrants who swim up the rivers and cross the skies in search of home.

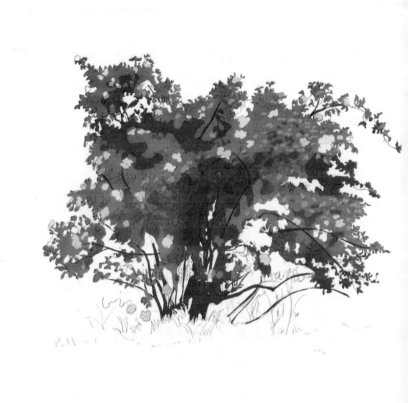

The Shape of Everything

In the summer of 2024 I spent hours in the garden cutting grass and strimming weeds. Raking dead leaves from under trees. Pruning branches and scraping ivy off the bark.

The funeral in Glangevlin had felt like the end of an era and left me with a sense of completion: that everything lives and dies in its own time and not a leaf falls but that God wills it. That there is a time for love and a time for sorrow, a time to be born and a time to die.

And it was as I cut dead wood out of the hedges one day that I noticed something on the grass; it was a cluster of petals that must have fallen in the previous weeks, and deep inside the hedge was a stem rising from the earth with leaves more oily than the dry green of other bushes. Tiny thorns like the fangs of a wolf ran like beads along the stem and I knew this was the old plant I had called my father's rose. A rose from Clare that passed half a century in Cavan and came to Leitrim thirty years ago. Now it had survived years of neglect and the voracious weeds that tried to choke it. It was still blooming.

I thought it would have been elegant to bring a little bouquet to my father's grave in Cavan, except that the flowers were all gone. But at least it focused me on making some gesture towards him.

The blessing of the graves at Killygarry where my parents are buried was scheduled for July the seventh.

On the day before the event I drove to Cavan with a shovel and hoe, and I brushed away the horsetail weed that grew through the grey pebbles and I placed small pots of begonia at each corner of the grave, and one large basket of begonia at the centre. Around me there were other graves in magnificent condition. Some with pebble stones as white as snow, and some with baskets of lilies and azaleas, and some dominated by stone carvings, enclosed by hedges and manicured little grass patches.

My parents' plot appeared humble enough among the grandeur of the dead, but the begonia blushed a deep red and it felt just right to me. I went home and returned the following morning.

Mass began at 11 a.m. though I did not attend, and outside the church the crowds were so vast and the line of cars on the side of the road so long that it took me a long while to reach the grave.

I walked up the incline past the little church and took a pathway through the city of burial plots and headstones presided over by white angelic figures in marble and limestone. Once again I came to the plot with the five red begonia plants, and to the black marble slab with the names: Nellie Finlay, July 2012, Michael Harding, July 1976.

And there I stood, in July of 2024.

It's a funny thing to say but when hundreds of people assemble in a graveyard, you would expect it to feel full. Yet graveyards are always empty spaces. I felt nothing as I stood listening to the prayers except perhaps the unusually chilly wind. A grave is a heap of clay and wood and bone. Nothing more. Even some of the lesser angels on top are made of plastic.

The prayers were said, the priest in his white robes moved as swift as a deer through the crowd, scattering holy water on graves to the right and to the left, and when it was over I drove towards Mullingar. I was due to share lunch with an old friend I had not seen for a few years and arranging it for the same day as the blessing of the graves was convenient.

We met in the Bloomfield Hotel and we both chose the roast beef but it was all gone so she settled for the bacon and I opted for turkey.

We chatted about horses and flowers, and the deaths of other friends we knew, and parents, and when we were leaving she remembered that she had a gift for me in her car. So we walked out to the carpark at the side of the hotel.

The gift was just a gesture of gratitude, she explained, since I was covering the meal. It was just something she had plucked spontaneously from her garden that morning. She opened the boot and there it was; a bouquet of pale pink roses.

A shiver went down my spine and goosebumps rose on my neck as if my father's hand had touched my shoulder with his faithful presence. It couldn't

I LOVED HIM FROM THE DAY HE DIED

have been a sweeter coincidence. It was the unintentional symmetry of the gift that mattered. And I felt the shape of him in that surprise – as a belonging, an unfolding, and as eloquent as a tiny rose.

I hope he felt the same in his dying: the mystical geometry of the universe unfolding in his death, like a cosmic rose, or an unexpected hand on the shoulder when all the leaves have fallen from the tree.

Acknowledgements

Thanks to my editor, Ciara Doorley, for her amazing support in the making of this book and the entire collection of memoirs.

Thanks to my brother, Brendan, for his encouragement and support over many years. To Gallery Press for allowing me to plunder a beautiful poem by Michael Hartnett for my title. Thanks to Simon, Helen, and Sophia for their love, to the cats, Charlie and Peabody, for their steadfast attention, to Louise Donlon for organising so many wonderful tours around previous books, to my cousin Michael Carroll for his friendship, and to the people of Glangevlin and the family of Joe (Mickey Oiney) McGovern and all his children.

And to my teacher, the Venerable Panchen Ötrul Rinpoche, and as ever to my beloved companion Cathy Carman.

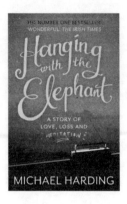

'In public or on stage, it's different. I'm fine. I have no bother talking to three hundred people, and sharing my feelings. But when I'm in a room on a one-to-one basis, I get lost. I can never find the right word. Except for that phrase – hold me.'

Michael Harding's wife has departed for a six-week trip, and he has been left alone in their home in Leitrim. Faced with the realities of caring for himself for the first time since his illness two years before, Harding endeavours to tame the 'elephant' – an Asian metaphor for the unruly mind. As he does, he finds himself finally coming to terms with the death of his mother – a loss that has changed him more than he knows.

Funny, searingly honest and profound, *Hanging with the Elephant* pulls back the curtain and reveals what it is really like to be alive.

Also available as an ebook

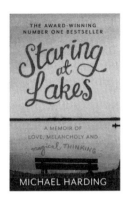

Throughout his life, Michael Harding has lived with a sense of emptiness – through faith, marriage, fatherhood and his career as a writer, a pervading sense of darkness and unease remained.

When he was fifty-eight, he became physically ill and found himself in the grip of a deep melancholy. Here, in this beautifully written memoir, he talks with openness and honesty about his journey: leaving the priesthood when he was in his thirties, settling in Leitrim with his artist wife, the depression that eventually overwhelmed him, and how, ultimately, he found a way out of the dark, by accepting the fragility of love and the importance of now.

Staring at Lakes started out as a book about depression. And then became a story about growing old, the essence of love and marriage – and sitting in cars, staring at lakes.

Also available as an ebook and audiobook

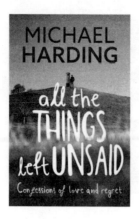

MICHAEL HARDING

all the THINGS left UNSAID

Confessions of love and regret

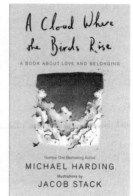

A Cloud Where the Birds Rise

A BOOK ABOUT LOVE AND BELONGING

Number One Bestselling Author

MICHAEL HARDING

Illustrations by

JACOB STACK

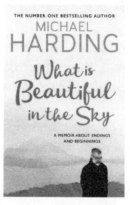

THE NUMBER ONE BESTSELLING AUTHOR

MICHAEL HARDING

What is Beautiful in the Sky

A MEMOIR ABOUT ENDINGS AND BEGINNINGS

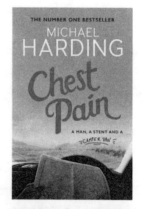

THE NUMBER ONE BESTSELLER

MICHAEL HARDING

Chest Pain

A MAN, A STENT AND A CAMPER VAN

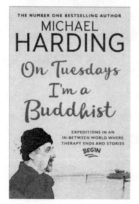

THE NUMBER ONE BESTSELLING AUTHOR

MICHAEL HARDING

On Tuesdays I'm a Buddhist

EXPEDITIONS IN AN IN-BETWEEN WORLD WHERE THERAPY ENDS AND STORIES BEGIN

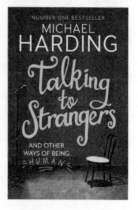

NUMBER ONE BESTSELLER

MICHAEL HARDING

Talking to Strangers

AND OTHER WAYS OF BEING HUMAN